The Autism & ADHD DIET

A STEP-BY-STEP GUIDE TO HOPE AND HEALING BY LIVING **GLUTEN FREE AND CASEIN FREE (GFCF)** AND OTHER INTERVENTIONS

Barrie Silberberg

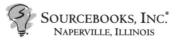
SOURCEBOOKS, INC.®
NAPERVILLE, ILLINOIS

Published by Sourcebooks, Inc.
P.O. Box 4410, Naperville, Illinois 60567-4410
(630) 961-3900
Fax: (630) 961-2168
www.sourcebooks.com

Library of Congress Cataloging-in-Publication Data

Silberberg, Barrie.
   The autism & ADHD diet : a step-by-step guide to hope and healing by living gluten free and casein free (GFCF) and other interventions / Barrie Silberberg.
      p. cm.
   Includes bibliographical references and index.
   1. Autism in children--Diet therapy. 2. Autistic children--Care. 3. Gluten-free diet. 4. Casein-free diet. 5. Parents of autistic children. I. Title.
   RJ506.A9S545 2009
   618.92'85882--dc22
                                    2008046040

Printed and bound in the United States of America
BG 10 9 8 7 6 5 4 3 2 1

This book is dedicated to my beautiful,
wonderful, and amazing son, Noah.
Because of you and your success with the GFCF diet,
together we are able to make a difference in the lives of
so many children with Autism Spectrum Disorders.

Contents

⇛ Acknowledgments ⇚

I would like to thank my parents, Blanche and Arthur Silberberg, who always believed that I could do anything that I wanted to do. To my beautiful, bright, precious, and very special daughter, Annsley Bella, whose smile, love, and encouragement always give me strength and provide me with joy. To my incredible, bright son, Noah, for just being yourself, and always shining and soaring above and beyond our expectations.

To my dear friend Mary Parker for showing me the inspiring magazine article, so many years ago, that helped me to help Noah receive his diagnosis, thus beginning our journey. To my uncle, Samuel Kohn, for reading my manuscript and helping me to edit it. To my wonderful agent, Neil Salkind, who believed in my passion and my message, who put up with my millions of questions so happily, and who quickly found me a publisher for this book.

To Julie, Melinda, Rachelle, Natalie, Joyce, Petra and Alex, Phyllis, Saswati, and Emma for taking the time to put your wonderful success stories into words for this book. To Alan Friedman, PhD, for your help and guidance with information about your peptide research. To Heather Gilliam, MPH, RD, for your dietary wisdom and words.

To Dave Morrison, PsyD; Gilit Gat, MA, ATR; Benjamin Kohn, OD; and Diane Mautner, MA, CCC-SLP (author of *Draw Me a Story*), for critiquing and assisting me with the therapy segments. To Shula Edelkind and Jane Hersey of the Feingold Association for assisting me in appropriately wording details of the Feingold Diet.

Thanks to Dave Morrison; Karima Hirani, MD, MPH; and all the others who've written endorsements for my book. Thanks to Donna Williams for writing the foreword and sharing with my readers about your success with the GFCF diet. Thanks to my editor, Peter Lynch, for all of his assistance and patience every step of the way. Thanks to Stephen O'Rear, my production editor, for seeing my manuscript through its journey.

Finally, to all of my friends who encouraged me, supported me, and had faith in me, who knew that I could do it!

⫸ Foreword ⫷

At six months old, my immune deficiencies began to manifest themselves through persistent infections and jaundice. By age two, in 1965, I drank bottles of (high salicylate) honey, cans of sweetened condensed milk, ate orange jelly and white bread with colored sprinkles, appeared deaf, showed no response to pain, and had self-injurious behaviors. A three-day hospital observation resulted in the label "psychotic." By the '70s, I ate boxes full of chocolate cookies and colored popcorn and ate flavored fluoride toothpaste (which strips the lining of the gut) from the tube. I was then labeled "disturbed." By the '90s I was diagnosed as autistic with a language processing disorder.

Around age ten, in 1973, I was introduced to complete meals and my three-year-old younger brother and I were put on zinc, vitamin C, and a multivitamin-mineral. He went from having six poorly pronounced words only understood at home to speaking in sentences two years later. I went from having around 10 percent receptive language to understanding half of most simple sentences and acquiring challenged-but-functional speech by age eleven. At first, I went and vomited my family's socially-invasive food, but then they hung a mirror on the living room wall and pushed me away from the dreaded table so I came to eat real meals with my reflection and the invasion factor was gone.

By my teens, I'd reverted to binge diets of doughnuts, chocolate bars, (high salicylate) nectarines and grapes, ice cream, and white bread, to the exclusion of all else—emotional blackmail of self starvation worked like a charm in controlling those around me so I could binge addictively on the foods which gave me drug-like effects.

By adulthood, my gut, immune, and metabolic disorders were all diagnosed—severe reactive hypoglycemia, B12 deficiency, white cell deficiency, no secretory IgA, gluten and casein intolerance, milk allergy (quickly followed by soy allergy), salicylate and phenol intolerance, a range of nutrient deficiencies, and food and chemical allergies. Next came what I called "The Dietary Wheelchair": a life of GFCF, low salicylate, low sugar diet in gaining and retaining as much language processing, visual processing, and management of mood, anxiety, compulsive, and attention disorders as I could.

I am often asked what degree health interventions played in the functioning I've achieved today. Certainly many of the often cost free or low cost interventions which helped me were not dietary, but dietary interventions contributed to around 50 percent of my improvements in information processing, communication, behavior, and relationships. As a result of these interventions, I didn't become non-autistic. I didn't lose my quirky, somewhat autistic personality. But I became less extreme, and that also meant I became less "autistic."

Not all people on the autism spectrum or with ADD/ADHD will have gut, immune, or metabolic disorders requiring a special diet, and even those who do may do so for quite different reasons. Just because we may share a diagnosis doesn't mean the underlying "autism fruit salads" are the same. There will be those for whom no dietary interventions work, those for whom GFCF doesn't work but low salicylate/low phenol does or who require both, those who only require dropping a particular allergenic food or who cope best off fried food or on complex carbs or even low carb diets. We are not all the same.

I have worked as an autism consultant with hundreds of people on the spectrum since 1997. Some of the children I've worked with had no health issues at all and many of the adults had things like social-emotional agnosia (inability to read facial expression or body language) or had personality traits which manifested "autistically" but did not have any signs of health related issues. However, some children who came to see me had allergy rashes, asthma, eczema, sinusitis, constant ear, nose, throat, and lung infections, and often they'd appear to have little receptive language processing, be uncoordinated, unable to visually track with their vision flitting from detail to detail as though they couldn't see things as a whole. Some would have easy bruising, "allergic shiners" (dark circles under their eyes), or were reported to have bowel problems. Some would display signs of marked mood, anxiety, and compulsive disorders and it was like being with someone on drugs. Although I'd also provide extensive suggestions on many environmental and social levels, far beyond focus on physiological issues, I'd often write reports asking their GPs to refer people for testing. Often parents would find it simpler to try thirty days of their child (or adults on the spectrum themselves) going GFCF/low salicylate/low sugar just to see if the effect seemed beneficial and to what degree.

I saw people after those thirty-day trials who had changed, sometimes dramatically, and occasionally saw those who had not changed at all. Some who'd appeared severely dyspraxic and uncoordinated were now observably less so. Some who were not toilet trained or had no speech had begun to babble and begun to use the toilet. Some who had been self-injurious or aggressive were less so or had ceased being aggressive at all. Some who had been unable to recognize and navigate visuals began to explore them and seemed to cope better with faces. Some who had had minimal speech and struggled to understand others now showed more interest in speech and were using their own more fluently. The autistic children and adults with gut, immune, or metabolic disorders who progressed through addressing these simply became better able to use the potential they already had. Helping those with gut, immune, or metabolic disorders to manage their health issues doesn't have to mean you fear difference or demonize autism.

The child of a dietician, Barrie Silberberg grew up around a sense of healthy diet. She has been through the journey of dietary interventions with her son, Noah, who is on the autism spectrum. Barrie has also watched this journey with many other families with children diagnosed on the autism spectrum and with ADD/ADHD. In this book she sets out clearly what dietary interventions are, who they might help, how they might help, the mental and emotional struggles in coming to terms with trying dietary interventions, and how to go about affordably implementing them. She includes an extensive list of products, stores, and websites related to dietary interventions as well as recipes, sample diet plans, and testimonials. Most importantly, she includes a vast range of other non-dietary therapies and approaches as part of a holistic approach which acknowledges that developmental disabilities require interventions on a range of levels. Her book is also a thought-provoking exploration of how modern society has come to accept dietary habits which are far from natural or healthy, the price we pay in making medications our first stop, and how families can embrace the sanity of sensible nutrition to logically improve the health of the gut-brain connection.

Donna Williams, Dip Ed, BA Hons
Author of the bestsellers *Nobody Nowhere*
and *Somebody Somewhere*
http://www.donnawilliams.net

≫ Introduction ≪

I have dedicated a large part of my life to healthy eating and staying away from chemicals, additives, and basically anything that is not natural. I grew up with a mother who is a registered dietician. She instilled in us the value of healthy eating; it was always part of our lives.

Chemicals do not taste good. Why force yourself to eat food that not only does not taste good, but is bad for you? There are so many additives, artificial ingredients, hormones, chemicals, preservatives, and other horrible ingredients—foreign substances with names we can't even pronounce, let alone understand what they could be doing to our bodies.

Do you wonder what effect these alien ingredients are having on our bodies? We have more cancer, more attention deficit hyperactivity disorder (ADHD), more autism, and more mental illness than ever before. We are not helping our bodies by feeding them unhealthy foods. Too many doctors just want people to "pop a pill." Too many so-called professionals and parents want a quick and "easy" fix. Way too many people are not watching what they consume or what they feed their children.

The old saying, "You are what you eat," resonates over and over again for me as I see what some of these foods are doing to our children. We all need to fight to remove toxins from our foods. We all need to pay attention to the foods we ingest and the effects they cause after they invade our bodies.

I am not dismissing the fact that there are many ailments that *do* require medication to change the imbalances in people's bodies. But look carefully at food, because a change in your and your children's diets could actually keep you off some medications. A change in food might make you feel and act much better and correct some of your body's imbalances.

You can make a change! This book can help you to change your lifestyle and eat healthier and safer foods. By reading it, you'll learn how to eat more appropriately with healthier foods, and how the suggested diet changes may be of particular value to children on the autism spectrum, as well as other disorders, and the members of their families.

Please consult with your child's or your own medical-care provider before starting this diet. To help you, consider contacting a practitioner pledged to support the Defeat Autism Now! approach of the Autism Research Institute. See the institute's website for more information: (http://www. autism.com/dan). Please make sure that you read the disclaimer on the website.

Defeat Autism Now! doctors specialize in working with children on the autism spectrum. They assist parents in helping to change their children's lifestyle by using dietary changes, supplements, and behavioral intervention. These doctors focus on healing the gut, ridding the body of yeast and other toxins, and possibly offering chelation and other interventions.

Consider going to a Defeat Autism Now! conference to learn more about their approach to helping children with autism spectrum disorders. For more information, visit http://www.defeatautismnow.com.

Finally, please read this book completely before starting the suggested gluten-free, casein-free diet. You'll need to understand many important topics before implementing and continuing the diet.

Chapter 1

⫸ Our Story, Our Miracle ⫷

Because of our son's miracle and the miracles of thousands of others worldwide who have experienced success with this diet and other interventions, I knew that I had to share our story and my knowledge, so that you, too, can achieve the success that we joyfully saw in our own lives.

When my son was in preschool, he played alone and only ate from a very select group of foods. He was very verbal, yet odd. I thought perhaps he was gifted. At age two, he taught himself the alphabet. At four, he taught himself to read.

Then, in kindergarten, my son's behavior was horrible. He threw things, screamed, and had uncontrollable meltdowns. He had severe sensory issues, very poor social skills, never changed his diet from peanut-butter-and-jelly sandwiches, macaroni and cheese, milk, cookies, crackers, chips, pretzels, yogurt, cheese, and french fries—and he had mushy stools. He had obsessions, but they were typical boy interests, like *Thomas the Tank Engine* and Disney movies.

When my son began first grade at a new school, he had a very difficult time. I kept researching websites about gifted children to find out why my son was different from other kids. Meanwhile, he continued to be in trouble constantly for inappropriate behavior. He was very violent and continued to have horrific meltdowns, and his sensory problems were causing him a lot of pain and suffering.

I brought articles that I found online to his teacher, showing her the odd behavioral traits and characteristics of brilliant children. They seemed to fit. But some aspects of his behavior did not fit and did not make sense. A multitude of questions kept running through my mind:

- Why can't he ever go outside without wearing sunglasses?
- Why does he run away from strong smells in the kitchen?
- Why does he always scream and cover his ears when he is around loud noises?
- Why does he eat mostly smooth foods and is so picky in his eating habits?
- Why doesn't he have friends like the other kids?
- Why is his interaction with other children not typical?
- Why does he always talk nonstop about certain things?
- Why can't he have a typical conversation, like his peers do?
- Why does he fall apart when his routine is changed?
- Why does he have severe meltdowns or crying fits whenever he is even slightly frustrated?
- Why can't he look anyone in the eye while speaking to them?
- Why doesn't he do imaginative play?
- Why is he so fearful of so many things?
- Why did it take him so long to be potty trained?
- Why are his poops never solid?

In the middle of my son's first-grade year, a friend of mine was reading a magazine. Inside was an article about a boy with Asperger syndrome (a form of high-functioning autism). She brought it to my attention immediately and said, "Read this. This is your son." She was aware of my son's odd and disruptive behaviors and knew that I needed answers.

I read the article and cried tears of joy and tears of sorrow. I was thrilled, because I had an answer. I knew this was what was wrong with my son. Yet, I felt sadness, because my son was autistic. I am still grateful to that friend who had the guts to approach me. She had one goal in mind: to help my son and to help me be able to help him. I am so glad that I was open to hearing this information and using it to give my son the help that he badly needed.

I called a student study team meeting at my son's school. When I mentioned the "A" word, all of the staff in attendance nodded their heads. They told me they had been discussing this and they, too, were fairly sure he was on the autism spectrum. The school counselor gave me several phone numbers to call and seek help.

This was the beginning of our road to autism—a long, challenging, yet rewarding road. With the help of the school psychologist, we were fortunate that my son received a diagnosis of autism from the California Regional Center system and thus became a client. This agency was able to provide and fund many services to help him on his way.

When second grade started, we had another team meeting at school to discuss my son's Individualized Education Program (IEP). His behavior was not improving, and the school did not want him there. He was incredibly disruptive in the classroom and on the playground. However, school officials were willing to have professionals observe him, allowing my son to try to prove that he could be fully included in a regular class-room. We agreed to meet again in November to decide what to do next.

Unfortunately, my son's behavior continued to be horrendous. He constantly was disruptive in class. Ever since my son's diagnosis, I had searched high and low to find answers regarding this thing called autism. One website that was extremely helpful was OASIS (Online Asperger Syndrome Information & Support, http://www.udel.edu/bkirby/asperger). OASIS was where I first read about the possible benefits of removing gluten (wheat, rye, and barley, as well as oats due to contamination) and casein (dairy protein) from a child's diet. It sounded insane, because glutens and caseins were all that my son ate. I told myself and everyone else that he would starve if I took away all of his favorite foods. What were these crazy people thinking?

My son's father (we are divorced) and I returned to school for my son's IEP meeting several weeks before the Thanksgiving holiday break. The director of elementary special education told us that our son did not belong in a regular, fully included classroom and not even in the Special Day Class. We were told that our son had to leave.

The appropriate environment for him, the team said, was a classroom for children with moderate to severe autism or a classroom for severely emotionally disturbed children. When the IEP meeting was over, we went to observe both of these classrooms. In the first room, we saw several nonverbal children who were stimming intensely (making rapid hand-and-arm movements). These children were being rewarded with dye-filled, gluten-filled cereal. Later I would gasp at the insaneness of this practice for children with autism spectrum disorders.

We objected, feeling that neither of these placements provided the least restrictive environment for our son. He was a very bright little boy with amazing verbal skills. Neither was the appropriate place for him, and we kindly told the director that our son would never be in one of those classrooms.

We decided that we had no choice but to try the ridiculous-sounding gluten-free, casein-free (GFCF) diet. With encouragement from several friends, we dove in headfirst. Over the four days of that Thanksgiving break in 2002, we removed dairy products from our son's diet. To our amazement and delight (and also that of the school's staff), our son was a much calmer child when he returned to school after the break. We saw *huge* changes in his behavior. So, we thought, if removing dairy could do this in basically four days, what could removing gluten do?

We removed gluten slowly at first and then permanently. The improvements were vast. The school personnel were shocked—and they allowed our son to remain in the regular classroom. I later discovered that food dyes and preservatives can also be disastrous culprits in causing inappropriate behaviors, so we stopped using all of them. I realized that, to achieve the best results, my son's vitamins, toothpaste, shampoo… *everything* had to be free of gluten, casein, dyes, and preservatives. None of these "pollutants" could be allowed to enter his intestinal system or touch his skin.

Our son's behavior improved dramatically. His sensory issues vanished. He was able to listen calmly to loud music, go outside without sunglasses, and sit in a room where onions were being cooked. It was a miracle. He still needed special services and time in the Special Day Class at his school, mostly to work on abstract writing and minor behavioral issues.

As I continued to educate myself on the GFCF Diet, cross-contamination issues, and the need to stay with the diet 100 percent, as well as with pollutant-free non-food items, our son kept improving bit by bit. He was calmer, happier, and more relaxed. His anxiety was gone, and he could engage in typical, everyday conversations about many different subjects.

Before the diet, every conversation turned into a monologue about his obsessions. He could not communicate back and forth with someone else, as people usually do in conversation. With the diet interventions, he began to communicate like a typical child. He later became fully included in his regular classroom, with no outside interventions from the school.

Since then, I have made the GFCF Diet my passion. I have dedicated my life to educating parents and professionals about the positive results possible when you change what goes into your body. The old saying, "You are what you eat," rings so true.

I have spoken about the diet at parents' meetings sponsored by our county autism society. I also have prepared a four-page starter guide to the diet and offered it to families all over the world via OASIS's message boards (http://www.udel.edu/bkirby/asperger), Yahoo Groups' GFCF Kids message board (http://health.groups.yahoo.com/group/GFCFKids), and Delphi Forums' celiac disease online support group (http://forums.delphiforums.com/celiac), as well as through other autism support groups. Through the years, many eager individuals have begged for my starter guide so that they, too, can experience the miracle that we have seen.

I wish everyone could see the changes that we have observed in our son. He has changed so much, due to the diet and to the wonderful behavioral service personnel who worked with him on social and behavioral skills. Everyone who knew our son in the early grades sees a totally different child today.

Some people might say that the school and outside interventions are what helped him. But I know, for sure, that the change is largely due to the GFCF Diet. My son has accidentally ingested gluten or casein several times, and each time the inappropriate behavior, meltdowns, and out-of-control craziness have returned. These behaviors often would take three days to appear and then three days to vanish and return him to normalcy.

A few years ago, our son made our family so proud. Fifth graders at his school, including our son, participated in the Drug Abuse Resistance Education (DARE) program, which ended with the students writing essays about what they had learned in the program. A DARE officer picked one essay from each of the three classrooms to be read at the final program by the student who had written it. That was three out of ninety-six students.

Imagine our joy and pride when our son's essay was picked! He received a ribbon, a medal, an award, and recognition for reading his essay to the other fifth-grade students and a room full of parents and school professionals. Many parents and staff members who had known my son in early grade school came up to me, shocked and pleased at how far he had come.

He had started at this school in a very different place than he was now. The school had gone from a place that didn't want him because he was too disruptive, too out of control, and did not fit in…to a place, years later, that rewarded him with honors for his greatness. Not bad for an autistic kid!

The following year, our son completed sixth grade at the middle school and received all A's in academics and all E's (excellent) in work habits and citizenship on his report card. In seventh grade, he took academic honors classes and earned B+'s or A's in all of his classes. He has come so far, and I know he will continue to soar!

He still has an IEP to assist with minor issues, one allowing the use of an assistive device to type his work (rather than painstakingly using pen and paper) and another allowing his teachers to make minor accommodations, such as giving him more time to complete assignments or permitting him to complete fewer problems per page.

He is still autistic. I do not deny that. Change of routine can still be a problem for him, as well as social interactions. But, to most onlookers, he appears to be a typical high-achieving student who handles honors classes well.

We know that our son has accomplished so much because of the change in his diet. I encourage you to follow the GFCF Diet with your child, so you, too, can achieve success and have proud and unforgettable moments.

Follow me to find out how to get started by changing the foods that your child consumes, how to follow through, and how to discover the light at the end of the tunnel. You are probably reading this because you see value in this idea. Stick with me, and I hope that you, too, will see how improving what your child eats can help you and your whole family live a brighter and happier future.

If you are skeptical or a nonbeliever, that is fine, too. Perhaps after reading this book, you will find the power, courage, and fortitude to try this diet and see for yourself that it can make a difference, probably without as much effort as you had thought.

So many parents of autistic children have questions that need answers. This diet seems difficult and perhaps impossible, yet it is much easier than you may think. Ask any parent whose child has followed the diet for at least six months, and you will hear phrases such as "a miracle," "vast improvements," "huge changes," "a different child," and "the best thing we have ever done." You'll hear, "My child spoke to me," "My child stopped hurting other children," "My child has calmed down," and many similar breakthroughs.

These parents will tell you how valuable the GFCF Diet is. They will tell you that it is not hard. It is not too expensive; and it is not overwhelming. Once these families got the hang of it, following the diet became part of their regular routine each day. When they saw the positive changes in their children, they realized that the time and effort they invested in implementing and continuing the diet were completely worth it.

I have written this book to give parents the will and the power to move forward and do what is in the best interest of their child or children. No one had written a step-by-step guide before this, but the information needs to be available, as the interest in, demand for, and knowledge of biomedical interventions continues to grow.

This book will answer many of your questions about the GFCF Diet and show you ways to make it work well for you and your family. There is no single best approach to following this diet or to doing any of the many interventions. Families choose to add interventions or not, to eliminate other foods or not, and to seek help from specialists or not. You will find examples in this book of approaches that families from all over the world have tried successfully.

Often success comes by trial and error. Many children have food allergies, in addition to intolerances, so they have to eliminate other foods besides glutens and caseins. This often throws parents into a tailspin over what to feed their children. But do not give up: there is so much hope, and the results will be so worthwhile for your entire family!

As the saying goes, "Knowledge is power." My goal is to provide you with the knowledge to make the right choices, do the right thing, and discover success along the way.

Chapter 2

❧ Before We Begin: First Ditch ❦ the Dyes, Preservatives, and Other Problematic Foods

Even though the gluten-free, casein-free (GFCF) diet does not specifically state that dyes and preservatives should be avoided, a lot of research suggests that putting artificial chemicals into a healthy, growing body is not a wise practice. I am including this information first, because I believe this is the first step in changing your child's diet.

I do not allow dyes and preservatives in my home. My personal experience, and that of millions of other parents, is that ingesting artificial dyes and preservatives in foods can have severe consequences, such as hyperactivity, anxiety, emotional upheaval, meltdowns, and skin conditions. Some reports even state that dyes and preservatives can cause cancer.

Understanding Dyes and Preservatives

What are dyes and preservatives, and why are they troublesome? First, let's take a look at dyes and artificial coloring.

Artificial coloring is classified in two categories: dyes and lakes. Dyes dissolve in water and are usually manufactured as powders, granules, and liquids. They can be found in beverages, dry mixes, baked goods, confections, dairy products, pet foods, and a variety of other products.

Lakes are frequently used in products that do not have enough moisture to absorb the dye or where the probability of dyes moving and changing would be an obstacle. Lakes are more stable than dyes and are used for coloring products that either contain fats and oils or lack sufficient moisture to dissolve dyes. Often lakes are used to coat tablets, in frosting on cakes and doughnuts, or in hard candies and chewing gum.

Dyes are often used in medications, both liquids and pills. They can even lurk in white or chocolate-brown foods that you would never suspect. Read the labels to become informed! Never guess about any food's contents without verifying its ingredients.

The U.S. Nutrition Labeling and Education Act of 1990 required labels on food packaging to protect and inform consumers by giving information about the food's ingredients and nutritional contents. The law stated that, as of May 8, 1993, these nutrition labels had to list all ingredients, including all certified colors, by name. In 1986, an advisory committee of the U.S. Food and Drug Administration (FDA) stated that Yellow No. 5 might cause itching or hives for a small population of individuals.

Preservatives are troublesome as well. Studies have found that some of the most detrimental preservatives for our bodies are: butylated hydroxyanisole (BHA), sometimes called E320 in other countries; butylated hydroxtoluene (BHT), or E321; and tertiary butylhydroquinone (TBHQ), or E319.

BHA and BHT are preservatives used to keep fats from becoming rancid. These preservatives can be found in many foods that families have in their homes, such as butter, meats, cereals, snack foods, ice cream, and vegetable oil. BHA and BHT are also used in non-food items, such as cosmetics, medicines, and more.

These preservatives are artificial antioxidants, also sometimes called synthetically produced antioxidants. They help food retain its normal color and appearance, rather than turning black or brown and decomposing.

(Do not confuse these chemically produced antioxidants with natural, food-based antioxidants, which are found in fruits and vegetables and play a healthy role in preventing chronic diseases and slowing the aging process in our bodies.) Foods treated with BHA and BHT last longer and are prevented from spoilage. But what are they doing to our bodies?

Evidence shows that some children and adults cannot metabolize these preservatives in their systems, thus causing health and behavioral irregularities. Studies have shown that these preservatives can cause allergic reactions, hyperactivity, rashes, and asthma. BHT (E321) has caused disorders in animals such as cancer, reduced body weight, and increased blood cholesterol levels, and has been linked to birth defects in rats. Many countries have banned these preservatives in their products.

For more information check out:
http://chemistry.about.com/library/weekly/aa082101a.htm
http://www.feingold.org/Research/bht.html
http://ntp.niehs.nih.gov/ntp/roc/eleventh/profiles/s027bha.pdf

Research and Studies about Dyes and Preservatives

There have been many important and troubling studies into the effects of dyes and preservatives.

In 1990, the FDA outlawed several uses of strawberry-toned FD&C Red No. 3 as a color additive. ("FD&C" designates this color as FDA approved to appear in food, drugs, and cosmetics.) The FDA banned the use of Red No. 3 in cosmetics and externally applied drugs, as well as the use of the color's non-water-soluble "lake." Research has shown that large amounts of this color caused thyroid tumors in male rats. Sadly, Red No. 3 is still used in foods and oral medications. You will find Red

No. 3 in maraschino cherries, bubble gum, baked goods, and a variety of snack foods and candy.

Research proved that FD&C Red No. 2 at a high dosage resulted in a statistically significant increase in malignant tumors in female rats. The FDA decided to ban Red No. 2 permanently because it had not been shown to be safe. However, Red No. 2 can still be found in Canada and Europe.

On September 6, 2007, a much-anticipated study on the effects of artificial dyes and preservatives on children was published online in the *Lancet*, a respected, peer-reviewed British medical journal. Psychology professor Jim Stevenson, PhD, and his team of researchers at the University of Southampton studied a group of children after they were given fruit juice, some of which contained a mixture of artificial dyes and the preservative sodium benzoate (E210–214 in other countries).

The randomized, double-blinded, placebo-controlled trial studied 153 three-year-olds and 144 eight- and nine-year-olds. The artificial colorings and the preservative being tested were removed from the children's diets during the time of the study. Parents and researchers kept daily diaries of the behaviors of the children being studied.

The findings showed that the children who consumed artificial dyes and preservatives clearly behaved more hyperactively when ingesting these substances.

To read more about this study, go to the University of Southampton's website (http://www.soton.ac.uk/mediacentre/news/2007/sep/07_99.shtml).

After the *Lancet* posted the story in 2007, the United Kingdom's national Food Standards Agency (FSA) decided it was time to make some changes. On April 10, 2008, the FSA recommended asking manufacturers to voluntarily remove six artificial colors by the end of 2009 and encouraged other European countries to follow suit.

Researchers found that if these dyes were removed, at least 30 percent of ADHD cases would vanish. These dyes also have been found to cause migraines, rashes, swollen skin, stomach upsets, water retention, asthma difficulties, and other allergic reactions.

Read more about this report:
http://www.food.gov.uk/news/newsarchive/2008/apr/coloursadvice

A 2002 study in the United Kingdom by the food firm Organix found artificial food colorings present in 93 percent of sweets, 78 percent of children's desserts, and 42 percent of milkshakes.

Many other countries have banned these dyes. They are inappropriate for all children, not just children on the autism spectrum or with ADHD. Our bodies do not need to ingest these toxins. We have choices of which foods we purchase, consume, and provide for our families. Shopping at healthier markets, ordering online, or shopping in the organic or natural section of your grocery store will allow you to purchase foods without these toxins. Healthier foods use fruits, vegetables, and other natural items for coloring, not chemicals.

Eliminating Dyes and Preservatives

How do you eliminate these toxins from your family's diet?

Start by eliminating all dyes and preservatives from your diet. You will need to read food product labels and not purchase anything containing dyes or preservatives. This will prepare you to start the GFCF Diet and help you get used to reading labels. Ridding your home of dyes and preservatives will introduce you to better tasting foods without chemical flavors.

The additives that should be eliminated are: synthetic dyes, artificial flavors, synthetic sweeteners such as aspartame, and three preservatives— BHA, BHT, and TBHQ. These dyes and preservatives are made from petroleum. There is no way for a consumer to know what goes into food as an "artificial flavor."

Salicylates are found in many wholesome, healthy foods, but these naturally occurring chemicals can be an irritant for some people. Foods that contain salicylates include apples, oranges, grapes, and tomatoes, among others. The Feingold Association provides comprehensive information on how to find replacements for foods containing natural salicylates and how to later reintroduce them. (More on this in Chapter 13.)

Reading Labels

To avoid harmful toxins and chemicals, you must learn to read labels carefully.

Reading labels is a very important and necessary process in this diet. You will soon become extremely familiar with reading and understanding labels on food products, medications, cosmetics, and hygiene products.

Dyes appear on labels with the name of a color, followed by a number, or with the word "lake" following the number. Often you will see "FD&C" before the color name. This stands for "food, drug and cosmetics," and indicates that this color is approved for all three uses. Only seven dyes are approved for use in foods in the United States, but many that have been banned from use in foods are still allowed in drugs and cosmetics. If the dye is not allowed in food, it is marked with just "D&C."

The most commonly used dyes in the United States are Red 40, Blue 1, and Yellow 5. In other countries, dyes often are spelled out as names, such as: Neutral Red, Allura Red (Red 40), Citrus Red No. 2, tartrazine (Yellow 5), Sunset Yellow (Yellow 6), Fast Green, Brilliant Blue (Blue 1), Gentian Violet, and many more.

Many countries identify dyes and preservatives by a numbering system. Each dye or preservative is assigned the letter "E," followed by a number, such as: E123, E104, E132, and so on. This is a confusing system, because it is difficult to remember which E's are harmful and which are harmless additives.

> For more information on the E–numbering system and how it relates to dye names, go to:
> http://www.feingold.org/E-numbers.html or
> http://www.ukfoodguide.net/enumeric.htm

The second thing to find on a label is anything listed as a preservative or chemical, such as monosodium glutamate (E621), aspartame (an artificial sweetener that can cause brain damage for people with high levels of phenylalanine, according to the FDA), nitrites or nitrates (E249–252), and sulfites (E220–228), all of which can have adverse reactions in many individuals.

Other Harmful Foods

We know that a number of other ingredients are just plain unhealthy for our bodies and should be avoided as much as possible.

Anything marked "artificial," for example, is not something you want to bring into your home. Artificial ingredients can cause many of the side effects that you are trying to eliminate. If any ingredient is listed as "artificial," put the item back on the shelf and move on. These ingredients are chemicals and are not good for your body.

Another ingredient that is best to avoid is high-fructose corn syrup (HFCS). HFCS is one of the reasons many of our children are obese. HFCS is a highly refined, intricately processed sugar substance made by turning cornstarch into a thick, clear liquid. Research has shown that

HFCS goes directly to the liver, releasing enzymes that inform the body to store the substance as fat.

Another concern in food is the chemical acrylamide. This is not listed in any ingredient list on food packaging, but it is something to consider when you are eating fried, roasted, or baked food. When a carbohydrate, such as a potato, is cooked at a very high temperature by baking, roasting, or frying, it produces acrylamide.

Researchers at the Swedish National Food Administration and the University of Stockholm discovered this in 2002. Since this survey, the FDA has begun to look into these findings and test acrylamide levels in foods. The FDA has reported that the discovery of acrylamide in food is a concern because acrylamide is a potential human carcinogen, based on high-dose animal studies, and is a known human neurotoxin. Further testing continues in this matter. (Research results are located at: http://www.cfsan.fda.gov/~dms/acrydata.html and http://www.cfsan.fda.gov/~dms/acrypla3.html.)

Reports have also been completed by the Food and Agriculture Organization of the United Nations and the World Health Organization. They state that acrylamide is known to cause cancer in animals. Also, certain doses of acrylamide have been found to be toxic to the nervous system of both animals and humans.

Once you have investigated these items and eliminated the potentially harmful ingredients from your pantry, freezer, refrigerator, and lives, you are ready to start integrating the GFCF Diet into your family's life. The next chapter gives you the basics of the GFCF Diet and tackles the questions you are most likely to have.

Chapter 3

⟫ Understanding the GFCF ⟪ Diet: Answering Common Questions

Children who exhibit some of the following signs and behaviors might benefit greatly from a gluten-free, casein-free (GFCF) diet. This diet eliminates gluten (wheat, rye, barley, oats [because of contamination], and a few other grains) and casein (protein found in milk or other dairy products). Often these children are diagnosed with an autism spectrum disorder (ASD) or attention deficit hyperactivity disorder (ADD/ADHD). These children frequently have problems, difficulties, or challenges such as the following:

- Focusing
- Loose stools
- Constipation
- Diarrhea
- Red ears
- Red cheeks
- Runny nose
- Night sweats
- Sleep disorders
- Eczema

- Sensory issues (bright lights; loud noises; strong smells; tags on clothing rubbing the skin; preferred textures, especially regarding food)
- Limited diet
- Refusal to try new foods
- Frequent meltdowns and inappropriate or extended crying fits
- Anger
- Anxiety
- Fear
- Violent behavior
- Difficulty with change
- Hand or arm flapping (called stimming)
- Head banging
- Walking on toes
- Lack of eye contact
- Obsessing over certain objects, subjects, or details
- Lining up toys or other items
- Poor social skills
- Playing alone
- Not interacting with other children
- Language difficulties or abnormalities
- Speaking very loudly
- Preferring much younger children, much older children, or adults over peers
- Acting as a policeman: giving orders to others or pointing out what they are doing wrong
- Difficulty understanding idioms
- Problems with following social cues or understanding jokes
- Eating mostly foods derived from dairy or wheat

Not every child with ASD or ADD/ADHD has all of these issues and traits, but many have a large number of them. If your child shows many of these traits but has not been diagnosed with ASD or ADD/ADHD, you might want to discuss your thoughts with your child's healthcare provider or school professional, or both.

Childbrain.com, a pediatric neurology website (http://childbrain.com/pddassess.html), offers a questionnaire that you can fill out, if you suspect any form of pervasive development disorder (PDD) in your child. These conditions can include autism, Asperger syndrome, childhood disintegrative disorder, Rett syndrome, and pervasive developmental disorder not otherwise specified (PDD-NOS).

A score of 49 or less on the questionnaire means no PDD; 50–100, mild PDD; 101–149, moderate PDD; and over 150, severe PDD. Print out and share the results with your child's physician. Ask him or her where you can go to receive an official diagnosis and for further assistance.

Regardless of the ultimate diagnosis, if at least ten of these symptoms fit your child, keep reading and consider trying the GFCF Diet with your child. Most parents are hesitant to try this new way of eating. I sure was. But guess what? I tried it, and the change in my son was tremendous.

Surely, you have many questions at this point, and it is important to discuss them up front. You are probably wondering:

- Why does eating these foods cause problems?
- How expensive is this going to be?
- Where can I find GFCF foods?
- Will my whole family have to change the way they eat?
- Why should we do this?
- How long will it take to work?
- Does it always work?
- If it does work, what changes can I expect to see?
- Won't my child starve?
- How long should we do this?

- What special arrangements should we make?
- What if our physician doesn't accept the value of the diet?
- Where do I begin?

Let's take a closer look at these common questions that parents have.

Why does eating these foods cause problems?

In the early 1980s, a number of researchers, including B. H. Herman, PhD, and Jaak Panksepp, PhD, studied urine samples from groups of autistic children. The urine of some of these children was found to contain two peptides, gliadomorphin and casomorphin, formed from incompletely broken-down proteins in gluten (found in wheat, barley, rye, and cross-contaminated oats) and casein (found in milk). In essence these children were behaving like morphine addicts.

In 1990, these findings were confirmed separately by Kalle Reichelt, MD, PhD, a researcher at the Pediatric Research Institute in Oslo, Norway, and by Paul Shattock, PhD, a British plant biologist and lecturer at the University of Sunderland and the father of an autistic son. Reichelt and Shattock found that 90 percent of the autistic children they observed had abnormally high peptide levels in their urine.

While working for Ortho Clinical Diagnostic, a division of Johnson & Johnson, chemist Alan Friedman, PhD, conducted a similar study using much more advanced equipment and aided by the use of mass spectrometry. Friedman confirmed the presence of the two peptides (not found in children on the GFCF Diet) in the urine of autistic children as well as two other opiate-like peptides, dermorphin and deltorphin, that were not found in the first two studies.

Many ASD children are suspected to suffer from a permeable intestinal tract, more commonly called a "leaky gut." When these children ingest foods containing gluten and casein, their intestines leak toxins that are absorbed into the bloodstream. These toxins work their way to the child's brain and bind to the opiate receptors. The gluten and dairy products that have been ingested, therefore, drug the child. The children react as if they are on morphine or heroin, creating behavioral disturbances.

These children are not having an allergic reaction, as much as showing an intolerance to these foods. They usually crave foods with wheat and milk, often exclusively. Their bodies require these foods like an addict requires his or her drug of choice. By almost exclusively consuming products containing gluten and milk, they also miss out on proper nutrition, because their diets exclude fruits, vegetables, and other important nutrients that the body requires.

> For more information on the effects of eating gluten and casein, please go to these sites:
>   http://www.glutensolutions.com/autism.htm
>   http://www.autisminfo.com/diet.htm
>   http://www.gfcfdiet.com/Explanationofdiet.htm

How expensive is this diet going to be?

This is often the main reason parents are hesitant to begin the GFCF Diet. They are so worried about the cost. I often respond, "What if your child needed medications or medical devices? Wouldn't you come up with the money to help him or her?" Changing your child's diet should not be treated any differently.

In fact, this diet is easier (even if it does not seem like it now) and possibly healthier than the way your children are eating now.

If you purchase foods that your child does not care for, many stores will let you bring back the opened package and get a refund. Whole Foods Market and Trader Joe's will always refund your money. Sometimes you do not even need the receipt, although they prefer that you have it with you. If you are in the store and are curious if your child will like the food, take it to Customer Service and ask if they can open the package and give your child a taste. If he or she likes it, you buy the package. If your child does not enjoy the food item, you do not have to pay for it. The food usually will not go to waste, because they often put it on display for customers to sample.

Remember, you can make many typical family meals that are naturally gluten free and casein free. Here are some examples of foods you can use:

- Chicken
- Turkey
- Other poultry
- Beef
- Veal
- Pork
- Lamb
- Fish
- Shellfish
- Eggs
- Corn
- Potatoes
- Yams
- Sweet potatoes
- Rice
- Quinoa
- Teff
- Millet
- Amarath
- Buckwheat
- Montina
- Beans
- Lentils
- Polenta
- Fruits
- Vegetables

Just make sure that any added sauces, condiments, toppings, spices, or other ingredients are also gluten free and casein free.

That said, the price you pay would be no different than for your regular purchases. You may think that your ASD child will not eat these foods. But in time, you will be surprised. After being on the diet for a while, you and your child will want to expand the repertoire of foods and he or she will be willing to try many new foods.

Encourage your children to try foods several times before completely ruling them out. Some experts say that you must taste a food as many as four times before you decide that you like it. Sometimes an enjoyable taste takes time to acquire.

Some GFCF packaged foods are more expensive than typical foods, but not always and clearly not often. Rather than buying packaged foods, you can go the cheaper route of making many meals and desserts from scratch. There are wonderful GFCF flours that you can purchase to make desserts. (More of this will be discussed in Chapter 5.)

Bread from Food for Life Baking Company costs around three dollars a loaf. A box of GFCF cereal is around two dollars. Ready-made frozen pancakes or waffles are about the same price as comparable wheat- and dairy-filled products.

Crackers, pretzels, and desserts can be pricier, but most store-bought corn tortilla chips and potato chips are gluten free and casein free. (To be safe, always contact the company by phone or email to verify ingredients.) Many desserts can be made from scratch. You'll also find that ready-made cookies in grocery stores are often more expensive than ready-made GFCF treats.

What can be costly at first is having to purchase extra cooking items—for example, cookie sheets, a toaster, a bagel cutter, pots and pans, a grill or griddle, colanders, and cutting boards—to be sure you are not cross-contaminating the GFCF foods from other foods that family members eat. When you are preparing GFCF foods, you will want to use only cooking items that you have labeled "GFCF." Labeling also will keep family members from accidentally using these items for foods containing gluten or dairy.

If you plan to use the same utensils to prepare GFCF foods and foods containing gluten and dairy, you must wash the GFCF items in the dishwasher to sterilize them and remove all proteins. If you do not own a dishwasher, use very thick dishwashing gloves, extremely hot water, and a clean dishrag used only for GFCF items. Having separate cookware and cooking items for GFCF foods is the smartest way to go. The risk of cross-contamination is too high and not worth it. (Cross-contamination will be discussed further in Chapter 6.)

Where can I find GFCF foods?

Health-food stores and specialty grocery stores, such as Whole Foods Market and Trader Joe's, are your best bet for specific GFCF foods. For a list of health-food stores worldwide, check out GreenPeople.org (http://www.greenpeople.org/healthfood.htm). Go to the website, and then scroll down to find your country (or state or province) and city.

More and more grocery stores are stocking GFCF foods. Many foods can also be purchased online. (Make sure that the foods you purchase are *both* gluten free and casein free.)

> Here is a list of some popular websites where you can order GFCF foods:
> http://www.allergygrocer.com
> http://www.glutenfree.com
> http://www.glutenfreemall.com
> http://www.glutensolutions.com
> http://www.kinnikinnick.com
> http://www.glutino.com
> http://www.glutenfree-supermarket.com
> http://www.ener-g.com

http://www.wellshirefarms.com
http://www.causeyourespecial.com
http://www.chocolatedecadence.com
http://www.choclat.com
http://www.sunflourbaking.com
http://www.amazon.com (under "grocery" or "gourmet foods")
To locate food brands and store locations that carry gluten-free, casein-free foods, go to GFmall.com (http://www.gfmall.com).
Additional websites for ordering and purchasing foods worldwide are listed in the Resources section at the end of this book.

Will my whole family have to change the way they eat?

No! As long as you take care to avoid cross-contamination, you can still have gluten and casein in your home. The most important thing to remember is that you must keep the foods separate. You will need separate shelves in the pantry and separate sections in the freezer or refrigerator.

I bought a small, used freezer at a garage sale so that my son has a place to keep his frozen foods. He knows he can eat anything in that freezer, and I don't have to worry about crumbs or drips falling onto his food. I also stopped baking with wheat flour. I only have gluten-free flour in my house. Flour does spread and fly, so keep this in mind if you choose to keep wheat flour in your home.

There is nothing wrong with having the whole family adopt this way of eating. The diet might help them as well. Some families make their home completely gluten and casein free, where everyone follows the diet. Family members have reported feeling much better after changing to the GFCF Diet. Some report feeling more awake, less fatigued, and freer of headaches, as well as being able to sleep better.

If the rest of the family is not going to follow the GFCF Diet, never exclude the child on the diet from special treats. We have a law in our home: we cannot eat anything that my son loved before the diet if we cannot find a suitable substitute for him.

Why should we do this?

In September 2007, a study was done at the University of Western Ontario in Canada, concluding that certain compounds produced in the digestive system are linked to autistic-type behaviors in laboratory settings, possibly demonstrating that what autistic children eat can alter their brain function.

What fascinated these scientists most was the fact that many of children on the autism spectrum craved breads and dairy products, causing many nontypical behaviors. One scientist in this study stated that he found a link between certain compounds that are producing bacteria in the digestive system. This bacteria produces propionic acid, a short-chain fatty acid, which in addition to existing in the gut, is commonly found in bread and dairy products, the very foods craved by so many children with ASD.

Many sources have shown that dairy and gluten cause opiate reactions in the brain. Thus ASD children have gastric abnormalities, severe issues, difficulty with change of routine, and cognitive functioning problems. These children also show immaturity; difficulty in communication skills, especially when it comes to crying fits; and many other traits not found in typical children, especially all at once.

The best reason to try this diet is that it might actually work. Your child might actually be on the path to greatly improving his or her condition. Your family, your child, his or her friends, his or her teachers, and others involved in your child's life may be able to see the real child hidden under the autistic umbrella, once this diet starts to work.

How long will it take to work?

Most people suggest following the diet for at least three months, with six months being optimum, to see if it works. This means three to six months of sticking to the diet 100 percent of the time. That comes after the trial and error involved in moving slowly onto the diet.

Why so long? The body needs quite some time to rid itself of the toxic effects that gluten and casein have caused. Also, you will need time to understand how this diet works, how it is to be implemented, and how to avoid cross-contamination. You'll also need to find ways to have your child accept the diet 100 percent of the time, especially when he or she is away from you.

You have to start gradually and work your way up to being 100 percent GFCF all of the time. (For those with celiac disease, you need to go 100 percent GF right away!) You will need a lot of time, knowledge, skill, and experience to achieve the most favorable results that everyone is seeking. Some children respond so well to the diet that their parents can see changes during the first week. However, this is not common for most children. Do not expect this outcome, but rejoice if you see changes quickly.

Does it always work?

Many skeptics refuse to believe that this diet works. There are parents who claim that they tried it and did not get the results they were expecting.

I truly believe that many negative outcomes occur for the following reasons: cross-contamination, not giving the diet enough time to work, not changing *everything*, not following the diet 100 percent, not altering non-food items (details on this later), and children cheating at school or at friends' or relatives' homes. One bite *will* make a difference. (Yes, Grandma, one tiny bite will hurt!)

That said, the GFCF Diet can and does work for many families who follow the details completely and fully. Succeeding with this diet takes guidance, patience, stamina, and the desire to do everything possible to make a difference.

If your child has been addicted to dairy and gluten products and you follow the GFCF Diet correctly, the changes will quickly become evident. The diet will work sooner, and you should see success. Doctors associated with Defeat Autism Now! say they see positive results from the GFCF Diet in 60–70 percent of their patients. Keep in mind that not all children with ASD are seen by one of these doctors, so success rates could actually be much higher!

If it does work, what changes can I expect to see?

If it works, you should start to see a new child emerge, like a butterfly hatching from a cocoon or chrysalis. Hopefully you will see a totally different, calmer, happier, and better adjusted child. You should see tantrums vanish or diminish. You should see most of your child's sensory issues improve or disappear.

Behaviors should improve. Fears, anxieties, depression, and meltdowns should improve or fade away completely. Stools should regulate to normalcy. The diet also should help in eliminating any gastric upset.

It should be time to celebrate. Others will notice and comment that they see changes in your child. Remember, the process takes many months. It will not happen overnight. It usually just gets better and better as time goes on. For those with celiac disease, you will see a huge change in gastrointestinal issues and a new path towards good health, as the body recovers.

Won't my child starve?

Gosh, we all think this. I sure did. After all, my son lived on milk, cheese, yogurt, ice cream, bread, pretzels, pasta, waffles, pancakes, cookies, crackers, cake, and other similar foods. He was a regular gluten-and-casein eating machine. I had no clue what I could do or how I could change his diet when these were the only foods that he ingested.

Little did I know that all of his favorite foods could be enjoyed on a GFCF diet. It took time, a lot of time, to find those foods. In the early 2000s, GFCF items were not as plentiful or available as they are today. I had to learn to be creative. I bought foods online. I made a lot from mixes or from scratch. But today, we see GFCF items popping up daily in many stores.

This is an exciting time to go GFCF. The shelves are filling every day with new, interesting, and, more importantly, delicious GFCF foods! No, your child will not starve. In fact, not only will he or she learn to enjoy this new repertoire of foods, but he or she also will begin to try new foods and actually like some! This may take years, but you can slowly incorporate new foods weekly or monthly, whatever works best for your child.

What special arrangements should we make?

Talk to everyone who comes in contact with your child—family members and friends; school personnel; daycare providers and nannies; religious personnel; sports team coaches and team parents; scouting leaders and parents; individuals involved with other extracurricular activities in which your child participates; and anyone else who will spend even five minutes with your child. Explain that your child should never consume anything other than what you provide for him or her. Explain that the items you provide must be kept in the baggie or container until your child removes them himself or herself. If any of these people take the food out of the bag for your child, they may have something on their hands to cross-contaminate it. Something airborne could fly onto your child's food, as well, so make sure your child takes care, too.

When your child is having a birthday or other celebration, you need to bring in your own goodies. Let all of the kids, not just your child, enjoy a GFCF and dye-free treat. This way your child can hand out the treats himself, if the teacher or coach allows it. Other kids need to see that your child's foods can and do taste great!

You'll also need a plan for dealing with other children's birthday celebrations. Start by asking your child's teacher for a list of all of the birthdays in the class. Mark your calendar at home with each child's birthday so you are prepared. Be ready to provide a treat for your child on that day so he or she is not left out when someone is celebrating a birthday in the classroom. Keep track of any parties or school activities, as well. Make sure your child is never without a treat that he or she can enjoy.

Many teachers pass out food treats as special rewards. Mention to your child's teacher that you will provide a box or bag of treats (toys, nonperishable foods, or GFCF snacks) to keep in the classroom. That way, the teacher can have your child pick from this box or bag when he or she is awarded a prize. Sometimes a teacher may even offer to purchase the treats. If so, make sure you give a detailed list of what is appropriate, and always check the items before your child gets a prize.

If your child has an Individualized Education Program or a Section 504 plan, make sure that the form states the correct information regarding your child's special eating requirements. Make sure that the emergency cards that are filled out at school and at other venues have GFCF and dye-free explained and highlighted for easy identification. The more information you provide, the better you can keep your child safe and sane.

Remember how hard it was at first for you to understand this new way of eating? Others will not understand to the extent that you do now. You can explain the details of this diet to other individuals, but that does not mean those details will sink in and be remembered. Be in charge. Be aware. Be involved, and do your best to educate and inform.

What if our physician doesn't accept the value of the diet?

Many physicians just want to prescribe medication. Unfortunately, medicines have many side effects and often just mask the problem. If you have followed the GFCF Diet strictly, imposed *all* other interventions, given everything enough time, and clearly still not had success, you might want to discuss medications with your physician, if absolutely necessary. Medications should never be the first thing you try.

Consider asking a Defeat Autism Now! practitioner, as mentioned in the Introduction, to assist you with biomedical intervention. What is the worst thing that could happen if you try the diet? Better yet, what is the best thing? The best thing could be a happier child and a happier family.

You could have a child who fits in with peers; a child who is calmer, more relaxed, more focused, less irritable, and less anxious; and a child who feels good in his or her own skin. The children who have had great success with this diet never want to go back. They feel too good with their new, improved body and self.

Where do I begin?

This is the pressing question. How do we start this new adventure? You undoubtedly are confused, perhaps angry, a bit anxious, clearly overwhelmed, concerned, and worried about starting this new endeavor. These are normal feelings. This is why this book was written—to provide a step-by-step guide to starting, maintaining, and continuing with little effort. The next chapter will walk you through the ins and outs of this really not-so-complicated diet.

Chapter 4

≫ Ready, Set, Go: ≪ Starting the GFCF Diet

First, take a deep breath and make sure that your attitude is up to par to start this new experience. Unless both parents—or whoever feeds your child—are on board together, positive results will not occur. When everyone is emotionally ready to begin, you will experience a win-win situation. That is probably the most difficult part.

If you are still reading, you must be ready to go—or perhaps continuing to read this book will give you the extra motivation and power to go for it. I have chosen to list the how-tos in a step-by-step format so that they are easier to follow and refer back to when you need to review this information.

> Always remember, companies change their ingredients. Never be afraid to call and inquire; in fact, it is a very wise thing to do.

Before you start, you should invest in a journal or notebook to keep detailed documentation of all of the foods that your child has ingested on a daily, if not on an hourly, basis. Write down where he or she ate the food, what it was, how it was prepared, what utensils were used, if he or she liked it, and any positive or negative reactions that you noticed. Also write down any non-food products that he or she has touched or that came in contact with any part of his or her body.

GLUTEN-FREE TRAVELING TEDDY BEARS

If you have a young or young-at-heart child (age three or older), you might want to consider ordering a Gluten-Free Traveling Bear when you are ready to start the diet. The Westchester Celiac Sprue Support Group in New York came up with the wonderful idea of providing a visit from a GF teddy bear for a child who must eat gluten-free foods. The bear visits were invented for children with celiac disease, but as long as you or your child eats gluten-free foods, you are welcome to invite a bear to visit your home for a few days.

Each bear has a GF grain name: Buckwheat, Teff, or Quinoa. They are cute, fuzzy friends, dressed in chef outfits and hats to bring comfort to children and let them know that they are not alone. Parents order the bears, using an online request form. The bear's visit costs $25, which is a tax-deductible donation to help the Westchester Celiac Sprue Support Group's efforts.

A teddy bear will be mailed to you to visit with you and your child. Your child may take the bear to school, on play dates, to groups or activities, or wherever your child goes. Having the bear can help him or her explain to other children about their new, specialized diet.

After about three days, you will be instructed to mail your bear to the next child to help comfort him or her. Parents pay to ship the bear to the next family. A map on the website shows all of the places that the GF bears have visited. Your town could be one of them! You might even be featured in the online memory book with your bear. A disposable camera is included with the package. You need to return a signed release form, if you wish to have your child's photo in the online memory book. These bears can be mailed all over the world. The website (http://www.westchesterceliacs. org/bears/bears.php) offers more about the bears, including the map of visits, parent information, a travel log, and a memory book.

Okay, you are now ready. Grab your highlighter to help you take notes, and away we go.

1. Get rid of dyes and preservatives in foods and non-food items.

This will give you needed experience in learning to read ingredient labels. (Refer back to Chapter 2 for more information on this subject.) You will be blown away by what you find written on package labels, especially in a typical grocery store. A huge list of ingredients, especially with some you have never heard of, is a definite warning sign.

At health-food stores or Whole Foods Market, you should never find anything artificial listed on the packaging. If you do, report it immediately to the manager. At Trader Joe's, about 98 percent of items are free of chemicals and additives.

Look for positive, healthy terms like "100 percent natural," "all natural," "organic," and "no GMOs" (genetically modified organisms) on the packaging to help you to make better choices with your grocery shopping. The word "natural" can be tricky. Many companies do a play-on-words with "natural," so look closely to see that the food really is 100 percent natural.

2. Change your child's personal hygiene and cosmetic products.

Many people do not realize that changing these items is as important as changing food items. When we think of the GFCF Diet, only food comes to mind. But clearly, for your child to become 100 percent GFCF and dye free, his or her toiletries also must be changed. Some sources state that contaminants can be sucked in through the skin. Some parents of children with autism have reported negative reactions caused by a non-GFCF product touching the child's skin. Others worry about these items coming in contact with the child's mouth and, from there, the intestinal tract. It is always better to err on the side of caution.

You will need to call the product manufacturer to be sure the product you use is safe from the toxins that you must avoid. You want these products to have no dyes, no preservatives, no gluten, and no casein (and no soy, if necessary). Labeling laws differ for food items and for cosmetics or personal hygiene products in terms of how ingredients are to be displayed on the label. (More on this in Chapter 7.)

A good brand of toothpaste is Tom's of Maine, available at Whole Foods Market, Trader Joe's, and many drug and discount stores. Stores often have a Tom's display showing the different flavors. Whole Foods Market has some Tom's flavors in the children's area of the toiletries section, separate from the adult toothpaste section. Check the box, because some Tom's toothpastes are fluoride free and others have fluoride added. Both types are GFCF and dye free.

All of Tom's products have great flavors like Silly Strawberry (with banana in it, too) and orange-mango for kids. Tom's of Maine also has grown-up flavors that are fine for kids. These flavors are: wintermint, peppermint, spearmint, cinnamint, apricot, lemon-lime, fennel, and cinnamon-clove.

The American Dental Association approves the fluoride type to help fight cavities. Some families prefer the fluoride-free type because they worry about the neurotoxins in fluoride. If you choose a formula with fluoride in it, make sure that your child spits the toothpaste out after brushing instead of swallowing it.

Tom's of Maine also makes soap, deodorant, and a few other products. Call the customer service departments of other companies to make sure the soaps, lip balm, lotions, creams, cleansers, moisturizers, dental floss, shampoos, conditioners, sunscreens, deodorant, and other cosmetics and products that you usually use are GFCF and dye free.

Some of these products have phenols and salicylates (more on these in Chapter 13), which could cause problems. Be aware that many lipsticks and other cosmetics have gluten in them. Most likely, they also contain dyes, so check around for more "environmentally friendly" makeup for your older female children. (Also, if your children get into your makeup you will feel safer.) Many cosmetic companies are manufacturing healthier, natural, and pure products.

Burt's Bees makes natural products, many of which are GFCF. Burt's Bees products are available online (http://www.burtsbees.com) and at many drug and discount stores, as well as health-food stores, in the United States. If you contact Burt's Bees, they can assist you in locating stores where their products might be available in other countries.

California Baby is another well-liked company that offers natural, GFCF, and soy-free products. These products are available throughout the United States at drugstores, discount stores, and certain supermarkets. California Baby products also can be ordered via the website (http://www.californiababy.com) and shipped all over the world.

3. Be aware of other non-food products.

You may be shocked to learn that many home and school products contain gluten!

Many stamps and envelopes use wheat substances in the glue section. Do not lick these items. Instead, use a sponge and be careful of the residue. Wash your hands completely with warm, soapy water after each use. Some stickers also have wheat on the glue side. Avoid skin and mouth contact.

Play dough often has gluten in it. Many such products have soy, too. You can order Colorations GFCF play dough through Discount School Supply (http://www.discountschoolsupply.com/Product/ProductDetail.aspx?product=7566) or Lakeshore Learning Materials (http://www.lakeshorelearning.com/seo/ca%7CsearchResults~~p%7C 2534374302091047~~.jsp/). Also, Crayola Model Magic and clay are GFCF. However, Crayola Dough contains gluten.

I do not believe ready-made, dye-free play dough exists. You can make some yourself, though, with natural dyes made from fruits and vegetables. (See the box.) Have your children wash their hands very thoroughly after playing with clay, Model Magic, or Colorations dough to remove any dye residue. Scrub their fingernails. Remember that the most common way for the substances to end up in their mouths is from their fingers. A better bet is for children to wear latex gloves or for you to make your own play dough from scratch.

Homemade Play Dough

- 1 cup rice flour
- 1 cup corn flour
- 1 cup salt
- 4 teaspoons cream of tartar
- 2 cups water
- 2 tablespoons vegetable oil
- food coloring—dye free, if desired

Put all of the ingredients into a saucepan on the stove. Cook over low heat for about five minutes, stirring constantly. The dough will be runny at first but will thicken as it cooks. Remove from heat. Cool to touch.

Knead dough on a flat surface to remove any lumps. (You may wish to wear disposable gloves to keep the dyes from coloring your hands.) Roll the dough into a ball and put it into an airtight container, and it can keep for months.

If you wish to make several different colors, divide the ingredients into parts before adding the coloring, set up several saucepans, and follow the directions specified above.

Call around to the manufacturers of items you use to find out if paints, markers, chalk, crayons, glue, glue sticks, paste, tape, face paints, Band-Aids, ink pads, and wipes are GFCF. For the most part, Crayola's products are GFCF, although the dough does contain gluten. Most of Elmer's glue products are GFCF, too. Always verify with the Customer Service departments of companies before using their products.

For up-to-date information on gluten-free arts-and-crafts supplies, go to Clan Thompson's Celiac Site (http://www.clanthompson.com/res_info_lists.php) and click on "Gluten-Free Arts and Crafts." Most likely these supplies also are CF, but call the company to confirm.

You will want to use dye-free laundry detergents, too. Call the company to verify that the product you use is GFCF. All or Cheer products contain no gluten, and both offer a dye-free, perfume-free formula. If your child has sensory issues, odor-free detergent is a very good thing. Other detergents also are GFCF and dye free. Some people have used and enjoyed these GFCF products: Shaklee, Seventh Generation, Arm & Hammer, and Melaleuca.

4. Be aware of other possible culprits.

There are other potential risks to be aware of, such as vitamins, dietary supplements, and medications.

Vitamins

Vitamins can be found at a variety of locations: Costco, drugstores, discount stores, Whole Foods Market, Trader Joe's, health-food stores, online, and at other retailers. Some brands that are GFCF and dye and preservative free are:

- Nutrition Now (Rhino)
- L'il Critters
- Solgar (KangaVites)

Trader Joe's has some GFCF varieties, too. Also check Kirkman Labs (http://www.Kirkmanlabs.com) for vitamins that can be ordered online. Look for the brands with many different types of vitamins all in one pill if your child is not eating enough of the right foods. Some vitamin pills contain a lot of sugar, so keep this in mind when choosing which to purchase. Some even have artificial sugars. Do not purchase these!

Dietary Supplements

Many varieties of dietary supplements can be ordered from Kirkman Labs (http://www.Kirkmanlabs.com), Houston Nutraceuticals (http://www.houston-enzymes.com/store), or Nutrition Now (http://www.nutritionnow.com/rhinosupport.htm#tablet) who makes Rhino pops (GFCFSF, dye and preservative free) with echinacea, vitamin C, and other vitamins. The company also makes chewable zinc and echinacea and liquid echinacea with vitamin C. Nutrition Now products are available at Whole Foods Market and some health-food stores. (More on supplements in Chapters 6 and 13.)

Over-the-Counter Medications

Finding over-the-counter (OTC) medications that are GFCF and dye free can be difficult, but they do exist. Luckily, Motrin and Tylenol have come out with a children's dye-free formula that is also GFCF. Caplets and capsules are another story. Many are coated with dyes, and often they contain gluten. Some parents prefer not to give Tylenol (acetaminophen) as it depletes the glutathione in the body. Many children with ASD have depleted glutathione already in their systems. Glutathione is a natural antioxidant.

CVS pharmacy keeps a list of OTC medicines that are gluten free, but you'll need to make sure they are casein free, which most are, and dye free, which many are not. CVS can be reached toll free at 1-888-607-4287.

Products change frequently, so make sure that you call before purchasing. Also, consider homeopathic formulas for coughs and colds. These products are available at Whole Foods Market or health-food stores. Always inquire about the ingredients.

Prescription Medication

Prescription medication can be tricky, as well. Before obtaining a prescription, have your physician contact a pharmacist to make sure that the medication he or she is prescribing is GFCF and dye free.

Unfortunately, finding a dye-free antibiotic is next to impossible. I would recommend at least asking your doctor or pharmacist for one that does not have Red 40. This dye usually causes the greatest amount of hyperactivity in children. Other dyes can be bad, but I think Red 40 is the worst in the dye category.

Doctors and pharmacists have lists of GF antibiotics and can make phone calls for you to the manufacturer. The Wheaton Gluten Free Support Group has an extensive downloadable list of GF medications and other medications to avoid because of their gluten content (http://homepage.mac.com/sholland/celiac/GFmedlist.pdf). You will be surprised. Contact a pharmacist to verify that the prescribed medication also is casein free. The Gluten Free Drugs website (http://www.glutenfreedrugs.com) also offers lists which contain some OTC medications.

Remember to contact the manufacturer to ask about a dye-free compound. Compounding pharmacies exist, but many medications are trademarked and cannot be formulated. A compounding pharmacy is similar to old-fashioned pharmacies where they would mix drugs from scratch and form the pills or capsules themselves. Compounding pharmacies still exist in many cities. You can still call a compounding pharmacist (under "Pharmacy" in your Yellow Pages) and ask for his or her suggestion and advice about what to do. Compounding pharmacies are also listed at http://www.iacprx.org or by calling 1-800-927-4227 to find one near you.

Often the pharmacist can recommend a different brand of medication or perhaps formulate it into a capsule that you can empty as needed. Or they can formulate the medication into a clear, dye-free, GFCF capsule that can be swallowed safely. (Do not ingest the dye-filled capsule.) Sometimes these pharmacists can compound liquid medicine, too. Keep the pharmacist's number handy in case your physician needs to contact him or her.

Cough and Throat Drops

Cough and throat drops often are not only full of dyes and other unhealthy items, but also loaded with sugar. Stick with Ricola brand cough and throat drops for children over age six. The drops come in a variety of flavors. They are 100 percent natural and contain herbs to help soothe sore throats. Do not buy the sugar-free products. They contain aspartame, which should be avoided because it is not a healthy choice for our bodies. Ricola herb throat drops are available in many drug and discount stores, as well as at Trader Joe's and health-food stores.

The Dentist's Office

The dentist's office can cause some concern. Almost everything dentists and hygienists want to put into your mouth could have gluten, dyes, or worse. Try bringing in your own toothpaste and demanding that they clean your and your children's teeth with that.

Some people will not allow fluoride in their mouths because of the neurotoxins it contains. If you have the dental hygienist use fluoride, pick a flavor that is dye free, such as marshmallow. Feel free to call the dentist's office before your appointment to ask for the fluoride manufacturer's phone number. That way, you can call ahead of time to verify that the fluoride and other substances are GFCF and dye free.

Chapter 5

≫ The Nitty-Gritty Part: Putting ≪ the GFCF Diet into Action

Now that you have some knowledge of easy items to remove from your child's diet, it is time to get serious about removing gluten and casein. That may sound overwhelming. But you can do it, if you take the right steps. And thankfully, many new foods are coming to stores daily to accommodate a GFCF lifestyle.

First, it is important to note that you should never go "cold turkey." (As stated above, those with celiac disease *must* go "cold turkey.") That would be too powerful of a jolt to your child's system. Your child has been acting as if he or she has been drugged. The toxins causing this can be painful, challenging, and detrimental to the body and the mind.

Your child's diet should be changed gradually over several weeks. Many children go through severe to mild withdrawal symptoms as you delete the toxins from their bodies. Remember, the leaky gut situation or abnormal gut flora act like a dangerous drug to the body as the toxins seep into the brain.

Some professionals who have studied autism and the GFCF Diet believe peptides cause an opiate reaction that may cause or trigger autism. Extracting toxins from the body is a serious matter. Not all children will have withdrawal or toxin die-off symptoms, but if you see these symptoms, do not be discouraged because they can be normal.

Withdrawal or toxin die-off symptoms can be behaviors such as acting as if in a fog, being cranky, having crying spells, exhibiting moodiness or anger, and more. If you are concerned, contact your child's physician. Never hesitate to call your practitioner. This is yet another reason to move forward slowly.

Let's take a closer look at the two steps in implementing the GFCF Diet:

1. Eliminating casein
2. Eliminating gluten

NEW LAW, NEW HOPE

On January 1, 2006, a new law went into effect in the United States. This law is the saving grace for those of us mandating a GFCF lifestyle. The Food Allergen Labeling and Consumer Protection Act (FALCPA—http://www.cfsan.fda.gov/~dms/alrgact.html) states that all packaged food products (except meat, poultry, and certain egg products) must list a warning if any of the top eight allergens appears in the product. These allergens are: milk, eggs, fish, crustacean shellfish, peanuts, tree nuts, wheat, and soy.

More than 160 foods have been identified as causing allergic reactions, but the eight foods listed above cause 90 percent of food-allergic reactions. These foods also cause many intolerances in people. Labels must now show the ingredients in plain language.

Companies that don't comply with this law are subject to civil and criminal penalties in accordance with the federal Food, Drug, and Cosmetic Act. The FALCPA applies to all packaged foods sold in the United States. If any food product is discovered to contain any undeclared allergens, the item will likely be subject to recall.

The package warning must include the word "contains" and then list the ingredients, if the food contains any of the top eight allergens. You will also see these phrases: "Manufactured in a plant" or "Made on equipment that processes" or "May contain traces of"...with the allergens listed.

Most people do not have a problem if the food-processing machines are sterilized and cleaned thoroughly. This statement protects the company. But if your child does react to products carrying that statement, you will want to avoid any foods that come in contact with the allergen. Take note that gluten is not in the top eight allergens, just wheat, which must be noted by law on the label if it appears in the product. So, barley, rye, oats, and the other non-GF grains will not be noted on a food product's label to warn you.

In August 2008, voluntary gluten-free labeling took effect. This effort has food manufacturers listing gluten content from wheat, barley, and rye, but not from oats. Food manufacturers also are required to test for cross-contamination. The legal allowed amount of gluten in a food product is 20 parts per million. This means that some products claiming to be gluten free may still legally contain a tiny amount. If you are uncertain about a product, call the company to verify the amount of gluten that it contains.

For international laws and regulations pertaining to allergens, see the World Health Organization-Food and Agriculture Organization of the United Nations' website (http://www.codexalimentarius.net/web/index_en.jsp).

How to Eliminate Casein

Usually the recommendation is to remove casein slowly from your child's diet first. Casein is the protein found in animal milk products, also known as dairy. These foods are milk from animals, cheese, yogurt, whey, butter, and lactose.

1. Read Labels to Avoid Foods with Casein

Check the labels of the products you buy. Caseinates and casein, both milk protein, must be listed on food labels by U.S. law. These ingredients usually are listed as "milk" on labels. Sometimes a milk protein is listed within parentheses, such as "(a milk derivative)." Note that a product with packaging reading "lactose free" or "dairy free" is not necessarily 100 percent casein free, but it could be. There are labels that can assist you in locating 100 percent casein-free products.

If you see the word "vegan" on a food package, for example, you know it is guaranteed to be 100 percent casein free. That's because individuals who live a vegan lifestyle do not consume any products with animal-related ingredients.

However, you do *not* have to limit yourself to products marked "vegan." Vegan means products that contain no animal milk products, no meats, no poultry, and no eggs. But while vegans do not eat eggs, they are completely acceptable on the GFCF Diet. Eggs are *not* dairy! Of course, if your child has an allergy or intolerance to eggs, you must avoid them.

Here's another helpful hint for you: when you are reading product packaging, look for the Hebrew word "parve," sometimes spelled "pareve" or "parev." This term means prepared without meat, milk, or their derivatives, in accordance with Jewish dietary laws. But this designation can still mean "contains a trace level of dairy contamination, under kosher law." So beware of this.

If you see the designation "P" on a package, this means that the product is kosher for Passover, something entirely different. It has nothing to do with being parve. Sometimes you will see a "K" for kosher on a product, accompanied by a "D," which means that the product *may* contain dairy. If you see this code, you will need to investigate further.

This could mean that the product was made in a factory that uses dairy or that the equipment might sometimes come in contact with dairy or that the machine did not go through a proper ritualized cleaning process, under kosher dietary laws. People who only eat kosher foods must consider this dairy, but on the GFCF Diet, if casein is not listed among the ingredient, you should be fine in consuming the product. Again, very sensitive people sometimes still have issues with products marked with the "D." If you are in doubt about what the designation means for that particular product, as always, call the company to verify.

Be aware also that some products have the word "whey" in their ingredient list. Whey is derived from dairy, so it should be avoided on the GFCF Diet.

2. Replace Milk with a Milk Alternative

Begin working milk out of your child's life slowly. I would suggest starting by giving your child 50 percent cow's milk and 50 percent of your chosen milk alternative. After a few days, if your child tolerates 50 percent of the alternative, change to 40/60, then 30/70, then 20/80, and so on, until your child is drinking 100 percent alternative milk all of the time.

Choosing a milk alternative is important. Many different types are available on the market. My favorite is Vance's Foods' DariFree, which is available in regular or chocolate flavors. Most people will tell you that, of all milk alternatives, DariFree tastes the most like cow's milk.

It is made from potatoes and is full of vitamins, minerals, and calcium. It also is free of all proteins, which are what usually give food its allergens. DariFree comes powdered, in round canisters. That makes it perfect for traveling and using when you need powdered "milk" in a recipe. This milk alternative only tastes good really cold, so mix it ahead of time and keep it in the refrigerator.

Vance's Foods is a really great company with a really good product. Ordering online from the website (http://www.vancesfoods.com) is recommended, because most stores do not carry DariFree, and if they do, it is more costly than ordering directly from the company. Products ordered online are usually delivered very quickly.

Other milk alternatives are made from rice, almond, other nuts, coconut, hemp, or soy. Many children have issues with soy products, so you should probably focus on non-soy products first. Later, when your child is fully 100 percent GFCF, you can reintroduce products with soy and look for unusual reactions. It may take a few days to notice a change.

Hopefully, soy will not be a problem because it is used in many foods, often as soy lecithin or soybean oil. Soy lecithin is used as a natural emulsifier and a stabilizer in many foods. It helps solidify foods such as margarine and helps keep chocolate from splattering while baking. Some people cannot tolerate soy protein, but they have no problem with lecithin or oil. This is something you will have to consider when experimenting to see if soy causes any issues.

Also, some rice "milks" contain barley, which is gluten, so check the labels or call the company to verify. Some rice milks even are labeled "gluten free" because they contain fewer than 20 parts per million of gluten, the legally allowed limit. Such products are not recommended for those who need to be 100 percent gluten free.

Milk alternatives can be purchased off the shelf at grocery stores. Some even come in 8-ounce containers, which are nice for traveling, or putting in lunch boxes, or using if you need just a small amount in a recipe. Some of these milk alternatives are also available in the refrigerated section of your grocery store.

Read the labels carefully because the amount of calcium, fat, protein, and sugars varies in these products. Try different types until you find what works well. Some people prefer chocolate or vanilla flavors. Again, try different types to see what suits you best.

Sometimes you might have to reintroduce an item a week or two later or have your child try the milk alternative several times before he or she starts to enjoy it and gets used to drinking it.

3. Introduce Cheese Alternatives

One of the hardest adjustments you will have to make concerns cheese. Sadly, none of the cheese alternatives tastes like cheese made with cow's milk. Some do not even melt well. They usually are decent and better tolerated if they are mixed with other foods.

You can find almond, rice, and soy cheese alternatives at many stores. These "cheeses" come in bricks and slices, but you will not find them sold with dairy cheese. Usually they are located where the soy and tofu products are found. Galaxy Nutritional Foods makes a vegan rice "cheese." Look for the purple vegan label, since Galaxy also makes rice cheese with casein.

Again, read the labels because many cheese alternatives contain caseinates and thus are not casein free. (Companies put the casein in these "cheeses" to help them melt.) Follow Your Heart makes several flavors of soy "cheese" that is vegan and does melt. However, wait before you introduce soy.

4. Adjusting Pudding and Yogurt

Other hard-to-adjust-to products are pudding and yogurt. Both are available in many flavors as soy alternatives. Tofutti Brands even makes soy "cream cheese" and "sour cream," in addition to cheese alternatives. ZenSoy makes GFCF puddings in several flavors. If soy is not a problem later, give these products another try.

Some puddings and yogurt are gluten free, casein free, and soy free (GFCFSF). Dr. Oetker, Ltd., makes a GFCFSF boxed pudding in many different flavors. You prepare the pudding by adding your choice of milk alternative and letting the mixture set in the refrigerator. Some milk alternatives set better than others.

Ricera Foods makes a GFCFSF rice yogurt in various flavors that is sold in the refrigerated section of grocery stores. In addition, Turtle Mountain, manufacturer of So Delicious casein-free frozen desserts, recently introduced a GFCFSF, coconut-based yogurt in several flavors.

5. Dealing with Margarine

Margarine also often contains soy. You can try to locate ghee, if soy is a problem. Ghee is a product from India and Egypt that you can often locate in Asian or Middle Eastern markets or in the Asian section of your grocery store. Sometimes you can find it in the refrigerated section.

Ghee is clarified butter that has been spooned off after cooking to avoid disturbing the milk solids on the bottom of the pan. The proteins, thus the casein, remain untouched at the bottom of the pan and are removed prior to packaging. Ghee is composed almost entirely of saturated fat, so it has a very oily appearance.

Coconut oil is another GFCFSF option. Two commonly used GFCF margarines are Earth Balance and *unsalted* Fleischmann's. Both do contain soy. Sometimes kosher stores carry GFCFSF margarines. Usually these kosher margarines are found near Passover time (March or April). The brand names are: Mother's from The Manischewitz Company or Migdal. You can call around to see who might carry these items. Unfortunately both brands contain hydrogenated cottonseed oil and preservatives, so these margarines are not very healthy or wise to use.

If you are baking, consider using vegetable oil, coconut oil, other healthy oils, ghee, or Spectrum organic shortening in place of butter or margarine in your recipes. To reduce fat and calories, and if apple-related products are not a problem, consider substituting 3/4 cup of applesauce and 1/4 cup of a healthy oil in recipes for baked goods that call for a cup of butter or margarine.

6. Introduce GFCF Ice Cream

Ice cream is a favorite food of many children and adults. You do not have to go without. New products have come on the market to help those on a GFCF Diet. The best tasting ice-cream alternative is Good Karma's Organic Rice Divine (http://www.goodkarmafoods.com). There are many terrific flavors! You can purchase these products by the pint, in small cups, or in bars. Good Karma does use a small amount of soy in its products.

Another brand of GFCF "ice cream," which uses nuts, is FreeZees (http://www.freezees.com). Five flavors—vanilla, strawberry, peanut caramel, fudge, and no-butter pecan—come in pints. All FreeZees products contain a small amount of soy. (Their Sweedee Pies frozen treats contain gluten, so do not buy them.) Tomberlies (http://www.tomberlies.com) makes a raw, vegan, GFCFSF, and egg-free "ice cream," but it is only available in stores in California and Las Vegas,

Nevada. Turtle Mountain recently introduced a line of coconut-based GFCFSF ice cream under its Purely Decadent label. It comes in five flavors. (More information is available at Turtle Mountain's website—http://www.turtlemountain.com/products/purely_decadent_Coconut_Milk.html.)

Think about making your own GFCFSF ice cream with an ice-cream maker. The book *Vice Cream*, by Jeff Rogers, has received rave reviews for recipes that you can use to make delicious, dairy-free "ice cream" from cashews. Whenever you make your own ice cream, make sure you use only GFCFSF ingredients.

For another option, try this recipe using Vance's Foods' DariFree powder and an ice cream maker:

Vanilla Vance's Ice Cream

- 9 tablespoons powdered DariFree (For a variation, use the chocolate powder to make chocolate ice cream.)
- 3 tablespoons tapioca starch or arrowroot
- 6 tablespoons sugar
- 3 cups water
- 3 tablespoons margarine, ghee, or healthy oil
- 2 teaspoons of vanilla extract or grated vanilla bean (Make sure extract is gluten free.)

Mix dry ingredients in a pot. Add the water, and turn on medium to medium-high heat. Whisk the mixture frequently to prevent clumping or sticking to the pan. When the mixture begins to bubble, add the margarine and vanilla extract. Stir until ingredients are dissolved, and remove the pot from heat. Refrigerate the mixture until completely cold. Add to ice-cream maker per instructions. Makes about a quart of ice cream.

A few companies make GFCFSF frozen dessert bars. One is Turtle Mountain with its Sweet Nothings, a fudge bar and a mango raspberry bar. Check with your store to see if they are stocked. More and more products are showing up daily.

Another option for something similar to ice cream could be dye-free, GFCFSF sorbets from Häagen-Dazs or Ben & Jerry's. If you go into a store, have them sterilize the ice cream scoop or get a new one. Tell them that your child is allergic to dairy. Both companies sell their packaged sorbets in grocery stores, as do Dreyer's-Edy's (Whole Fruit Sorbet), Sharon's Sorbet, and Ciao Bella.

How to Eliminate Gluten

Now that you know what casein is, how to avoid it, and how to substitute for it, let us move to gluten.

1. Go Slowly

Gluten may be harder to manage than casein, but you will be shocked and pleased at how many ingredients and different types of "flours" you can incorporate into the GFCF Diet. We seem to be surrounded by breads, cake, cookies, crackers, muffins, pretzels, and more. Yes, GF-floured products will be difficult to find if you are eating out, unless you go to a GF-friendly restaurant, bakery, or store. But for this chapter, let us focus on eating at home.

Just like going casein free, you should go slowly in changing over to being gluten free. (Unless you have celiac disease.) Studies have been proven that children need to try a food up to ten times before they decide they like it. The average adult has 10,000 taste buds coating the surface of their tongue. Children have even more, with some even dotted along the inside of their cheeks. This is why there are so many young, picky eaters and why, as we grow older, our tastes often change and our repertoire of foods grows.

Purchase a few highly recommended GF products and introduce them to your child. If your child does not like them, put them aside to try again later or return the product to your store. Most stores will happily refund your money, no questions asked, and you do not even need to present a receipt. Always ask about the store's return policy before purchasing a gluten-free item for the first time.

2. Understand How Many Foods Contain Gluten and Need to Be Avoided

Gluten is found in many grains that are typically considered staples in most homes. Gluten can be defined as wheat, barley, rye, oats (from cross-contamination), and other more unusual grains such as spelt, triticale, bulgur, durum, semolina, couscous, and malt. You can find a detailed list at the Celiac Sprue Association's website (http://www.csaceliacs.org/gluten_grains.php) that tells you which grains and flours do and do not contain gluten.

Sometimes on food labels, gluten is listed as modified food starch, natural flavoring, or hydrolyzed vegetable protein (HVP). You also may find gluten hidden in many luncheon meats, sausages, and hot dogs. (Gluten is often used as a stabilizer in these foods.) Turkeys often are injected with HVP as part of the basting process. Avoid all self-basted poultry for that reason.

In the United States, the manufacturer must list on the food label whether wheat was used in making a food product. But often gluten lurks as an anti-caking agent. Foods might be dusted with wheat on processing lines, or it may be mixed with dried fruits to prevent sticking or clumping. Read the labels. Call the company. Soy sauce is one item made with wheat that seems to surprise most people.

3. Purchase Only Gluten-Free Products

The best way to avoid gluten is to eat only gluten-free products. Searching for GF foods has become easier, because one out of 133 people is being diagnosed with celiac disease and, therefore, needs a GF diet. Many people also suffer from dermatitis herpetiformis, a skin rash disorder caused by an allergic reaction to eating gluten. Add the ASD families now changing to a GFCF style of eating, and there is quite a need for companies to produce a greater variety of GFCF foods. Not only a variety, but tasty and delicious foods.

To give you an overview of the best products available, let's review the top brands listed by people who eat GF foods. "Different strokes for different folks" comes into play in choosing GF products because some people enjoy some of these foods more than others. Your selections will depend on taste, flavor, texture, and other preferences. Check the websites provided here to locate where these products are sold near you or to order them online. (More brand names for other products are listed later in this chapter.)

Food for Life Baking Company

One of the most favored bread brands seems to be Food for Life (http://www.foodforlife.com). The bread is available in many varieties: raisin pecan, rice almond, rice pecan, white rice, brown rice, Bhutanese red rice, and China black rice. Food for Life also offers yeast-free multigrain bread and several varieties that are yeast and soy free—millet, fruit, and seed medley; whole grain, brown rice; and white rice. Many people also enjoy Breads From Anna, which are gluten-free bread mixes. You have to use a bread-maker or bake the mix in the oven. (More on this in Chapter 6.)

Kinnikinnick Foods

Kinnikinnick Foods (http://www.kinnikinnick.com) makes wonderful GFCF foods, many of which are available at Whole Foods Market and at health-food stores. If a store does not have what you want, but you see it on the company's website, ask the bakery manager if he or she can order it for you. Remember to look for the symbol designating the Alta GFCF product line on Kinnikinnick foods. Every product the company makes is gluten free, but not all are casein free.

The product list on the Kinnikinnick website displays a green (does not contain) or red (contains) box under each product posting. These symbols explain which foods are free of which allergens or additives and which contain allergens or often-to-be-avoided ingredients. The eight most common ingredients that people try to avoid (casein, yeast, sugar, soy, eggs, corn, nuts, and potatoes) are listed with each product.

Besides their great breads, the company makes doughnuts, cookies, cinnamon rolls, pizza crust, English muffins, bagels, hot dog and hamburger buns, cereal, waffles, muffins, and a few other items. Keep in mind that not all Kinnikinnick products show up in stores. Again, ask the bakery manager if he or she can order what you want. That way the store will pay for the shipping, not you, and the store wins because it will have a customer for life! You also can order directly from the Kinnikinnick website for a flat fee of ten dollars to cover shipping costs.

Ener-G Foods

Ener-G Foods (http://www.ener-g.com) has manufacturing lines that are guaranteed to be wheat free, gluten free, dairy free, peanut free, and tree-nut free. The processing plant also is a kosher-certified facility. Ener-G has great products such as a loaf, not called bread because the U.S. FDA and the Canadian Food Inspection Agency informed them that calling a product "bread" meant that it had wheat in it. Other companies do not follow these regulations.

In addition, Ener-G offers crackers, pretzels, cinnamon rolls, cookies, brownies, doughnut holes, doughnuts, cake, English muffins, pizza shells, hamburger and hot dog buns, dinner rolls, rice pasta, snack bars, and a variety of GFCF flours, baking needs, and egg replacer powder.

Ener-G products that are GFCFSF include: Wylde pretzels, chocolate-chip snack bars, and chocolate chips.

Gluten-Free Pantry

Gluten-Free Pantry (http://www.glutenfree.com) wins hands down for having the best brownie mix. Even the name, Chocolate Truffle Brownie Mix, makes your mouth water. The company specializes in gluten-free mixes and has many different types. Unfortunately, some of the mixes contain dairy, and some have soy. Read the labels, and when in doubt, call the company.

Namaste Foods

Namaste Foods (https://www.namastefoods.com) makes several excellent GFCFSF mixes for cakes, brownies, cookies, pizza crusts, muffins, and waffles or pancakes. Namaste products are free of gluten, casein, soy, tree nuts, corn, potato, and peanuts. You can buy them in stores or online.

Enjoy Life Natural Brands

Enjoy Life Natural Brands (http://www.enjoylifefoods.com) offers a variety of foods that are free of gluten, casein, soy, corn, peanuts, tree nuts, eggs, fish, and shellfish. They have great cookies, snack bars, chocolate chips, bagels, trail mix, and granola. You can find them at Whole Foods Markets and other stores, as well as through online retailers such as Gluten Free Mall.

Tinkyada

Food Directions makes Tinkyada rice pasta (http://www.tinkyada.com), by far the best GFCF pasta, many celiacs agree. Tinkyada does not get mushy like so many other GF pastas and comes in eighteen different shapes and forms. This is truly excellent pasta, and many people cannot distinguish the difference between it and wheat-based pastas.

EnviroKidz

Nature's Path Foods' EnviroKidz product line (http://www.envirokidz. com/food) includes great kid-friendly cereals and rice bars. Gorilla Munch cereal has corn as its main ingredient and is GFCFSF. The cereal is shaped like tiny balls. Peanut Butter Panda Puffs cereal is also corn based and shaped like tiny balls. However, it contains soybean oil and thus is not soy free. Koala Crisp cereal is GFCFSF. It is rice based, with cocoa added, and is shaped like puffy rice.

Amazon Frosted Flakes cereal is GFCFSF and made from corn. The shapes are like typical corn-flake cereals. Leapin' Lemurs cereal is GFCF (contains soybean oil) and has both chocolate and peanut-butter balls. It is made from corn. Beware: some EnviroKidz cereals and waffles are not gluten free!

Among the crispy rice bars, the berry- and peanut butter–flavored bars are GFCF but may contain soybean oil. (Do not eat the chocolate bars, because they contain milk.) Nature's Path also makes EnviroKidz GFCF vanilla animal cookies that do contain soy. Note that only the vanilla cookies are GFCF.

Glutino

Glutino Foods (http://glutino.com) makes a wide array of gluten-free foods, yet not all are casein free. Some of their breads are GFCF, but many are only GF. Some of their products also contain soy. Read the labels. Besides bread, Glutino makes French toast, pretzels, crackers, hard breadsticks, "O"-shaped cereal in honey-nut and apple-cinnamon flavors, pasta, and cookies, some of which have milk and thus are not casein free. Glutino also makes apple, blueberry, chocolate, and cranberry breakfast bars that are GFCFSF, although other Glutino bars are only GFCF.

Ian's Natural Foods

Ian's Natural Foods (http://www.iansnaturalfoods.com) makes GFCFSF, allergy-free products, as well as products containing wheat and milk. Read the labels. Look for the red ribbon on the front of the packaging that designates an allergy-free food. Ian's makes chicken nuggets, chicken patties, fish sticks, lightly battered fish, popcorn, turkey corn dogs, onion rings, french fries, Alphatot alphabet-shaped potato puffs, French toast sticks, and full meals. You'll find them all in the grocery freezer section. Ian's also makes boxed, individually wrapped cookie buttons. Note that the chocolate-chip buttons are not CF or SF, and the cinnamon buttons contain soy. Recently, Ian's came out with do-it-yourself pizza kits and pasta kits that come in a canister and can be found on the shelves in stores. They continually come up with more and more allergen-free products.

Van's International Foods

Van's International Foods (http://www.vansintl.com) makes GFCF waffles, as well as those with milk and wheat. Read the front panel on the box. Make sure you see the green triangle in the upper-left corner that designates gluten free. All of the GF waffles are vegan, so you know they are also casein free. However, the waffles are made with soy flour. They come in a variety of flavors: buckwheat (which is gluten free), blueberry, apple cinnamon, flax, and original.

Foods by George

Foods by George (http://www.foodsbygeorge.com) makes GFCFSF English muffins, brownies, pizza crust, and biscotti. However, these foods are only sold east of the Mississippi.

> Bars are a favorite quick snack, and several companies make GFCF varieties. (Read the label, because some contain soy.)
> Some favorites, besides those already mentioned:
> • Larabar and Jocalat bars (https://www.larabar.com/secure/index_.php)

- Bumble Bars (http://www.bumblebar.com)
- Arico bars and cookies (http://www.aricofoods.com)
- Clif Nectar Bars (http://www.clifbar.com). Read the labels, because not all Clif Bar products are GFCF.

Bob's Red Mill Natural Foods

One of the best friends that you will find in the GFCF world is Bob Moore, of Bob's Red Mill Natural Foods (http://www.bobsredmill. com/gluten.php). Bob has a huge assortment of GF flours and related products. These include: tapioca flour, sweet rice flour, brown rice flour, white rice flour, buckwheat flour, amaranth flour, millet flour, fava bean flour, black bean flour, almond meal flour, potato starch, potato flour, cornstarch, flaxseed, garbanzo bean flour, sweet white sorghum flour, green pea flour, quinoa, and rice bran flour. Bob also has a variety of mixes and other items used for baking. He even carries GFCF oats.

Authentic Foods, Shiloh Farms, Gluten-Free Pantry (owned by Glutino Foods), and Arrowhead Mills are a few other companies that manufacture GFCF flours and baking mixes. Check out ethnic markets, listed under "Grocers" in the Yellow Pages, where you often can find reasonable GFCF flours for your pantry.

Now that you know who makes these great flours, you probably are wondering what you can do with them. Your other new best friend is Bette Hagman, affectionately called the gluten-free gourmet. Mrs. Hagman, who passed away in 2007, was the guru of GF cooking and baking. One of the first things that you should do in starting this diet is to grab a Bette Hagman cookbook. You may want to glance at a few first at the library and then decide which of her many books to purchase.

Soon after Mrs. Hagman was diagnosed with celiac disease, she began to live in her kitchen, experimenting with hundreds of flours and ingredients to create recipes for foods that taste like the real gluten-based food that she and so many others loved. She mixed 1/2 cup of bean or corn or rice or tapioca or potato starch or flour and 1/4 cup of another flour or starch with a pinch of this and a pinch of that to create tasty meals, side dishes, and desserts—all gluten free. You can adjust her recipes as needed to prepare GFCF or GFCFSF items.

Mrs. Hagman also created recipes for dry-ingredient mixtures to keep on hand for later use. Using these mixes, you simply add wet ingredients, mix, and cook or bake, making meals or desserts faster and easier to prepare. Her company even packages some of her flour combinations for purchase to save time for cooks and bakers.

Some of her flours should be kept in the freezer or refrigerator, while others do fine on the pantry shelf. I always figure that freezing the flours extends their life, as well as the taste. This is especially true if you do not use the flours frequently.

Here is a chart to help you learn about many of the flours that Bette Hagman used in her cookbooks.

FLOUR	BEST USED FOR	STORAGE
White Rice	cakes, cookies	in pantry
Brown Rice	bread, crackers	refrigerator or freezer
Garbanzo Bean	bread, cake	refrigerator
Garfava Bean	bread, cake, cookies	in pantry
Soy	fruited cakes, cookies	refrigerator
Sorghum	cakes, cookies, breads	in pantry
Arrowroot	cornstarch alternative	in pantry
Cornstarch	mixes	in pantry
Potato Flour	mixes	buy fresh
Potato Starch	mixes	in pantry
Sweet Rice	thickening	in pantry
Tapioca Starch	fruit dishes, mixes	in pantry

By combining her flours in special ways, Bette Hagman created many wonderful mixes that can be used as dry ingredients for her recipes. Here are a number of these flour mixes, taken from page 28 of her book, *The Gluten-Free Gourmet Makes Desserts*, that you can make and store for later use.

Gluten-Free Mix (aka GF Mix)   For 9 cups of mix
Store in dry cupboard.

2 parts rice flour	6 cups
2/3 part potato starch	2 cups
1/3 part tapioca starch	1 cup

The GF Mix is often used to make cake, cookies, pies, waffles, pancakes, and breads.

Featherlight Rice Flour Mix (aka Featherlight Mix)   For 9 cups
Store in refrigerator or freezer.

1 part rice flour	3 cups
1 part tapioca starch	3 cups
1 part cornstarch	3 cups
1 tablespoon per cup potato flour	3 tablespoons

The Featherlight Mix is usually used to make cake, pastries, and cookies. It can be purchased premixed by Authentic Foods.

Light Bean Flour Mix   For 9 cups
Store in dry cupboard.

1 part garfava bean flour	3 cups
1 part tapioca starch	3 cups
1 part cornstarch	3 cups

The Light Bean Flour Mix is used to make breads and muffins.

Four Flour Bean Mix	For 9 cups
Store in dry cupboard.	
2/3 part garfava bean flour (Authentic Foods makes this.)	2 cups
1/3 part sorghum flour (Red River Milling makes this.)	1 cup
1 part tapioca starch	3 cups
1 part cornstarch	3 cups

Four Flour Bean Mix is used to make pancakes, waffles, cookies, and cakes. It is available premixed by Authentic Foods.

Bread Flour Mix	For 9 cups
Store in refrigerator or freezer.	
1 part white rice flour	3 cups
1 part brown rice flour	3 cups
2/3 part potato starch flour	2 cups
1/3 part tapioca starch	1 cup

Bread Flour Mix is used to make bread.

Flour Mix Chart from the book *The Gluten-Free Gourmet Makes Dessert* by Bette Hagman. Copyright © 1999 by Bette Hagman. Reprinted by permission of Henry Holt and Company, LLC.

GFCF Brands by Food Type

Always check the labels when considering brands of GFCF foods, because some manufacturers also make products that are not GFCF. Most of these products state on the package that they are gluten free, casein free, or both. Keep in mind, too, that manufacturers often change their ingredients. If you are in doubt about a product's ingredients, call the company.

Also, while some of these brands are only available in certain parts of the United States or the world, most can be ordered online. Online sites are listed throughout this book, as well as in the Resources section at the end of this book.

Note that some food products of Gluten-Free Essentials contain artificial ingredients and dyes, so please verify the ingredients before purchasing this company's products. All other brands listed should be free of dyes and preservatives. However, some of the items listed here contain soy. Please read the labels carefully if you are avoiding soy and other ingredients.

Breakfast Foods
- Cereal: Nature's Path EnviroKidz, Glutino, Enjoy Life Natural Brands, Nu-World Foods, U.S. Mills (Erewhon and New Morning brands)
- Cinnamon rolls: Ener-G, Kinnikinnick
- Waffles: Van's (not all are GFCF), Trader Joe's brand
- ·French toast: Glutino, Ian's
- Pancakes: Trader Joe's brand
- Pancake and waffle mixes: Authentic Foods, Bob's Red Mill, Namaste, Orgran Natural Foods, The Cravings Place, 1-2-3 Gluten Free, Gluten-Free Essentials, 'Cause You're Special, Arrowhead Mills

Breads/Tortillas
- Bread: Food for Life, Kinnikinnick, Ener-G
- Bread and muffin mixes: Whole Foods Market's 365 brand, The Cravings Place, 1-2-3 Gluten Free, Gluten-Free Essentials, Gluten Evolution's Breads from Anna, 'Cause You're Special
- Hot dog or hamburger buns: Kinnikinnick, Ener-G
- Bagels: Kinnikinnick, Sterk's Bakery
- Pizza shells or crust (ready-made): Kinnikinnick, Ener-G, Sterk's Bakery
- Pizza crust mix: Chebe Bread Products, 'Cause You're Special, Arrowhead Mills, Namaste

- English muffins: Kinnikinnick
- Doughnuts: Kinnikinnick, Ener-G
- Tortillas: Trader Joe's (brown rice), Food for Life (brown rice and corn), La Tortilla Factory (teff wraps)

Snacks
- Chips: Terra Chips, Lundberg Family Farms, Arico Cassava chips (Also some other store brands—check with the company about cross-contamination.)
- Pretzels: Ener-G, Glutino
- Crackers: Glutino, Ener-G, Glutano
- Snack bars: BumbleBar, Arico, Larabar, Jocalat Bars, Enjoy Life, Clif Bar, Glutino
- Chewing gum: Verve's Glee Gum
- Marshmallows: Golden Fluff Snacks' Elyon brand, Pangea Vegan Products

Meals and Main Courses
- Chicken nuggets: Wellshire Farms, Ian's, Bell & Evans (black box), Martha's Homestyle
- Hot dogs: Applegate Farms, Shelton's Poultry
- Lunch meat: Boar's Head Provisions, Applegate Farms, Wellshire Farms, Hormel Foods' National Choice products, Shelton's
- Corn dogs: Wellshire Farms, Ian's
- Sausages: Wellshire Farms, Applegate Farms, ATK Foods' Sausages by AmyLu (not all flavors are CF), Trader Joe's (some), Aidells Sausage Company (not all GF and some not CF)
- Bacon: Wellshire Farms, Applegate Farms, Hormel Foods' Natural Choice
- Frozen dinners: Ian's (some), Amy's Kitchen (some)
- Pasta: Food Directions' Tinkyada brand, Trader Joe's, Orgran, DeBoles, Mrs. Leeper's, Riso Scotti's Pastariso brand, Glutino
- Cheese alternatives: Galaxy Nutritional Foods' Vegan brand rice

cheese, Follow Your Heart's soy "cheese," Galaxy's Soymage soy "cheese"
- Yogurt: Ricera Rice Yogurt, WhiteWave Foods' Silk Soy brand, Stonyfield Farm's O'Soy brand, WholeSoy & Company, Springfield Creamery's Nancy's Soy brand, Turtle Mountain's So Delicious brand

Desserts
- Sorbet: Sharon's Sorbet, Häagen-Dazs, Ben & Jerry's, Dreyer's-Edy's, Ciao Bella
- Popsicles: Whole Foods Market, Trader Joe's, Minute Maid, Cool Fruits' Fruit Juice Freezers
- Ice cream: Good Karma, FreeZees, Imagine Foods' Rice Dream brand, Turtle Mountain's Soy Delicious brand, Tofutti, Tomberlies
- Ice cream cones: Gluten Free Foods' Barkat brand
- Pudding mix: Dr. Oetker's, Morinaga Nutritional Foods' Mori-Nu Mates
- Ready-made pudding: ZenSoy
- Cookies: Enjoy Life, MI-DEL Cookies (some), Nana's Cookie Company (some), Ener-G, Glutano, EnviroKidz (some), Pamela's Products (some), Kinnikinnick, Josef's Gluten Free, Orgran, Arico
- Graham crackers: Josef's Gluten Free
- Cake, brownie, and cookie mixes: Namaste, Gluten-Free Pantry, Bob's Red Mill, Pamela's Products, Authentic Foods, Whole Foods Market's 365 brand, The Cravings Place, 1-2-3 Gluten Free, Gluten-Free Essentials, Cherrybrook Kitchen, 'Cause You're Special, Arrowhead Mills
- Pie crust (ready made): Kinnikinnick
- Pie crust mix: 'Cause You're Special, Gluten-Free Pantry, Authentic Foods
- Frosting mix: Cherrybrook Kitchen
- Chocolate sauce: Ah!Laska, Wax Orchards
- Candy and cake decorations: See Chapter 6.

For more brand names than are listed here, to specify a certain type of food, or to find out what products can also be soy free, corn free, rice free, potato free, nut free, egg free, sesame free, yeast free, or sugar free, go to AllergyGrocery.com (http://www.allergygrocery.com/search.php). You'll see a checklist of ingredients that you may want to avoid, such as gluten, dairy, soy, and peanuts. You also can specify acceptable Feingold Stage 1 or Stage 2 products. Put a checkmark next to each ingredient that you do not want in the foods you purchase. Then click on "Search now" to see brand names of products that will work for you.

For additional brand names available outside the United States, see the websites listed under the heading "Eating Outside the United States" in the Resources section. The countries are listed in alphabetical order, so just look under the name of the specific country you want.

Other GFCF Diet Programs

You will soon discover there is not just *one way* to implement this diet, but many different approaches, styles, and choices. I recommend reviewing some of the great websites out there to familiarize yourself with many of the food items that are acceptable and those that are not. These sites also offer extensive information regarding the diet, including steps for putting it into practice for your family. A few websites to start reading are:

- Autism Network for Dietary Intervention (http://www.autismndi.com)
- GFCF Diet Support Group (http://www.gfcfdiet.com)
- Talk about Curing Autism (http://gfcf-diet.talkaboutcuringautism.org)

Of course, hundreds of other sites address gluten-free and casein-free diets and foods. All you have to do is search for "GFCF," and they will come up. However, I feel the three mentioned above are the most comprehensive, informative, and detailed.

Chapter 6

❧ Buying and Preparing ❧ GFCF Foods

One of the most frequently asked questions about the GFCF Diet is: "Where can I buy these special foods?" This chapter will address that important question, as well as another: "How do I prepare these foods?"

Buying GFCF Foods

You can try to shop for GFCF foods in the specialty sections at your local grocery store. For the best selection, however, go to a specialty store, such as those listed below, or order online. Ask if the store will give you a discount if you order in bulk. Often stores will give you 10 percent off the regular price if you buy their products by the case.

Let's look at the best specialty stores for purchasing GFCF products.

Whole Foods Market

Whole Foods Market (http://www.wholefoodsmarket.com) has more than 275 locations throughout the United States in thirty-seven states and the District of Columbia, in Canada (Ontario and British Columbia), and in several locations in the United Kingdom. More stores are being opened all the time. Whole Foods provides a list of its GFCF foods as part of a list for special diets (http://www.wholefoodsmarket.com/specialdiets).

Trader Joe's

Trader Joe's (http://www.traderjoes.com) is always introducing new GFCF food items. (Again, read the labels for soy.) They carry GFCF pancakes, waffles, cookies, granola, bread, bagels (Midwest), rolls (Midwest/East Coast), bars, candy, fruit leathers, desserts, brown rice pasta, and some other household staples. The company also is constantly expanding its store locations. Currently, Trader Joe's stores are in twenty-three states and the District of Columbia. Trader Joe's also offers a list of gluten-free foods (http://traderjoes.com/labels_and_lists.html) but no casein-free list.

Wegmans Food Markets

Wegmans Food Markets (http://www.wegmans.com) has seventy-one stores in New York, Pennsylvania, New Jersey, Virginia, and Maryland. Two to three new stores open every year within those five states.

Amazon.com

One of the largest selections can be found online at Amazon.com (http://www.amazon.com, http://www.Amazon.ca, or http://www.Amazon.co.uk). If you do order from Amazon using one of these websites, please go to this link first to connect to Amazon: (http://www.aspergersyndrome.org/bookstore.html). A portion of the costs will go directly to help run OASIS's message board for children with Asperger syndrome or high-functioning autism and families. OASIS volunteers receive no other compensation, except from private donations.

Amazon lists gluten-free foods under "gourmet foods" and "grocery." Usually, if you spend twenty-five dollars or more, shipping will be free. Look at these websites for coupons for dollars off at Amazon and other online retailers: (http://www.currentcodes.com or http://www.naughtycodes.com; you can also do a search for "coupon codes").

Other Resources

Many other specialty-food websites offer a variety of allergy foods online. Many of these sites have been listed in Chapter 3. Some of these sites allow you to check off boxes of the allergens that you need to avoid. A list will then pop up with all of the products that match your dietary needs.

Many people order their foods online from a variety of sources. If you plan to do so, compare prices for the items, as well as the shipping charges, to make sure you get the best deal. More resources and websites are listed in the Resources section at the end of this book, including where to purchase or order food internationally.

Examining Foods for GFCF

In purchasing foods, you may find that you cannot determine whether or not an item is GFCF. Checking with the company itself can be useful. Many larger corporations will mail or email you a list of their GF products. This will give you a head start in checking to see if those products are also CF and SF, if needed. Some items will be obvious. For example, if cheese is in the product's name, of course the product is not CF.

Most companies will assist you via phone or email if you need more help in deciphering the ingredients in their products. Here are links to contacts at some of these major companies:

- Nestlé USA: http://www.nestleusa.com/Public/ContactUs.aspx or 1-800-225-2270
- Frito-Lay: http://www.fritolay.com/fl/flstore/cgi-bin/contact_us.htm or 1-800-352-4477 (USA) or 1-800-376-2257 (Canada)
- Kraft Foods: http://kraftfoods.custhelp.com/cgi-bin/kraftfoods.cfg/php/enduser/ask.php or 1-877-535-5666
- General Mills: http://www.generalmills.com/corporate/contact_us/contact_us.aspx or 1-800-248-7310

- Seneca Foods: http://www.senecafoods.com/contact.shtml or 1-315-926–8100
- Del Monte Foods: http://www.delmonte.com/contactus/Contact. asp or 1-415-247-3000
- Pinnacle Foods: http://www.pinnaclefoodscorp.com/public/ contact/index.htm or 1-973-541-6620
- Dole Food Company: http://www.dole.com/CompanyInfo/ Contact/ContactUs.jsp or 1-800-356-3111
- Campbell Soup Company: http://www.campbellsoup.com/faqs. aspx or 1-856-342-4800, ext. 2225
- ConAgra Foods: http://www.conagrafoods.com/utilities/customer_ service.jsp or 1-877-266-2472
- Boar's Head Provisions: http://www.boarshead.com/contact.php or 1-941-955-0994
- Hormel Foods: http://www.hormel.com/templates/othersites/ contactUs.asp or 1-800-523-4635

Preparing GFCF Foods

When you are preparing GFCF foods and planning your child's diet, you'll want to keep these important factors in mind:

- Cross-contamination
- Compensating for "lost" nutrition, especially:
  - Calcium
  - Protein
  - Fiber

Cross-Contamination

One of the most important rules while following the GFCF Diet is to avoid cross-contamination (CC). I cannot emphasize enough how important this is.

Cross-contamination occurs when your hands or a utensil touch something that contains gluten or casein, or both, and then your hand or that utensil touches your child's GFCF foods. You have just contaminated the GFCF items with the foods that you must avoid. Another, more common form of CC occurs when the GFCF food comes in contact with a tiny crumb or a tiny drip of gluten- or casein-containing food. That can then set off your child's diet and cause undue stress for the whole family, especially the child. This can occur via a toaster, a pan, a bagel cutter, or a cutting board. It can also occur if you wipe your hands using a dish towel that has gluten or casein on it or touch the counter top, an appliance, or the cupboard where contaminated products have been. If you have wheat flour and other products containing gluten or casein in the home, these products can fly and contaminate your GFCF foods. Never allow anything with gluten or casein to come in contact with the GFCF foods. Never means never!

Avoiding cross-contamination in the products you buy is important as well. Some manufacturers cannot promise that they keep their equipment and manufacturing areas clean of gluten or casein or other allergens. A company spokesman might say, "We cannot promise that CC has not occurred." But you will not know this unless you contact the company and ask. Some newer companies specify that their products are manufactured on dedicated equipment or in a dedicated facility. This means that they only manufacture GF, CF, or GFCF products, whatever they claim to make.

To avoid cross-contamination in the home, think about the cookware and supplies you use in the kitchen: colanders, cutting boards, pots, pans, grills, griddles, cookie sheets, cupcake tins, blenders, mixers, food processors, can openers, silverware, spoon rests, ice-cream scoops, plastic straws, measuring cups and spoons, graters, dishrags, sponges, cleaning cloths, and towels. You must remove any physical trace of gluten or casein from the surface of these items. Put them in the dishwasher or washing machine, as appropriate, or buy new ones and mark them "GFCF only." Keep these new items in a separate area so no mistakes are made and they are kept safe from CC. Even in the dishwasher, food particles often remain stuck. Always look on every plate, utensil, and bowl to make sure that gluten or casein residue is not left. When in doubt, wash the item again in the dishwasher. Keep in mind that some surfaces—such as wood, stoneware, Teflon, and cast iron—are porous. They absorb food particles that can remain under the surface and then transfer gluten or casein into your food. Avoid these utensils.

Here are some tips for avoiding cross-contamination in your home:

- Never use the same knife in the margarine, mayonnaise, peanut butter, or jelly that has touched any gluten or casein product. This means you need two sets of these and similar spreadable foods— one for those eating foods with gluten and casein and another for those on the GFCF Diet. Label them clearly so mistakes never happen! Another option is to buy squeeze bottles. You can often find these for condiments. Just make sure that the spout never touches a gluten or casein surface.

- Buy a separate toaster. Mark it clearly so that no one puts anything with gluten into it or even near it. If you are going to be away from home, you can remain safe by purchasing toaster bags to toast your bread in the toaster or use on the grill. These bags keep the bread from touching the contaminated surfaces. Order from Celinal Foods (http://www.celinalfoods.com/store/index.php?categoryid=1 18&productid=17) or other GFCF online vendors.

- Buy a separate bagel cutter. Keep it far away from anything resembling gluten or casein. Mark it so only GFCF products will touch it.

- Keep foods containing gluten or casein far away from GFCF foods on tabletops or countertops.

- Keep separate ice cube trays. Crumbs and drips can easily stick to the ice.

- Keep separate bags of chips, or pour some chips into small bags to keep gluten or casein-touched hands away from the bags. Mark them clearly. (Some chip manufacturers have cross-contamination problems because their equipment is not cleaned properly after coming in contact with dairy or gluten. Contact the companies, if you are concerned.)
- Use parchment paper on cookie sheets to avoid cross-contamination. Throw the paper out when you are finished using it.
- Wash your hands with hot, soapy water if you have to touch both types of foods or items containing gluten or casein. Keep wipes handy for little hands and countertops. Remember, food particles can remain under fingernails, too. Better yet, touch the GFCF foods first and then the non-GFCF foods.
- Keep the floor clean for those who might be crawling around on it. Crumbs and spills could get into a young child's mouth this way.
- Keep toys belonging to your child on the GFCF Diet separate from others and, if possible, sterilize the dishwasher-safe toys in the dishwasher. Gluten or casein could easily be transferred from a toy onto the hands and then into your child's mouth.

Pay attention to what you are doing. Do not beat yourself up if you make a mistake. You are new at this, so you will need time and practice to get it right. Do not be rushed; just do your best to look around your kitchen and think before you act. Soon, the diet requirements will come naturally, and you will get the hang of it.

When you are eating at restaurants or at friends' homes, take time to educate the people involved. One time, for example, I was ordering for my son at a popular burger restaurant. I explained to the young man behind the counter that my son was allergic to wheat and could not eat the bun. He informed me that the bun was "white," not wheat.

One lady from the celiac disease forum suggested saying, "He cannot have bread or anything like that because he has a food allergy. Nothing can touch the plate, so please do not just take a bun off if you make a mistake." This is imperative to mention. Croutons or buns cannot simply be removed from a plate and then your child's food placed on it. Remember one crumb or one sip means cross-contamination and the possible return of traits, behaviors, or health problems that have vanished or improved.

Compensating for "Lost" Nutrition

Because you are removing foods that provide nutritional value from your child's diet, you might be concerned about how to replace these vitamins, minerals, proteins, and calcium in his or her diet. There are supplements (as mentioned in Chapter 13) and other ways to replace these valuable nutrients. Please discuss this with your doctor or a registered dietician.

Beyond supplements, though, you can find healthy alternatives to replace missing nutrients in your child's diet.

Calcium

The lack of calcium seems to worry parents the most because it is in all of the dairy products that your child used to consume. Our bodies store more than 99 percent of their calcium in our bones and teeth, helping to make and keep them strong. The remainder goes throughout our bodies in the blood, muscle, and the fluid between cells.

Calcium helps our muscles and blood vessels contract and expand, secreting hormones and enzymes and sending messages through the nervous system. The National Institutes of Health states that children ages one to three years old should consume at least 500 milligrams of calcium a day. Children ages four to eight should consume 800 milligrams, and children nine to eighteen, 1,300 milligrams.

There are many healthy ways to include calcium in our diets without drinking or eating dairy products. Dark green vegetables contain a decent amount of calcium, but children may not want to eat them—or to eat enough. Some great vegetables for calcium are:

- Collards: One cup has 357 milligrams of calcium
- Kale: One cup has 179 milligrams of calcium
- Broccoli: One cup has 178 milligrams of calcium
- Okra: One cup has 176 milligrams of calcium

Another method of getting calcium into your child's body is to have him or her drink calcium-fortified juices, which often have as much as 300 milligrams of calcium per cup. To find out how much calcium these juices contain, read the labels. In the nutritional facts table, you will see calcium listed as a percentage. A listing of 30 percent means 300 milligrams, 20 percent is 200 milligrams, and so forth. Vance's DariFree, as mentioned in Chapter 5, has 300 milligrams per cup.

Soymilk has 300 to 400 milligrams of calcium per cup, making it a good alternative if your child can tolerate it. Rice and almond milk have less calcium, but they still do have some, while most coconuts milks do not contain any calcium. Hemp "milk" has 460 milligrams of calcium per 8 ounces.

Several calcium supplements are on the market. L'il Critters makes chewy gummy bears that have 125 milligrams of calcium each. (Be aware of the sugar content, if these pose an issue.) Calcium also can be purchased in powder form from health-food stores or Whole Foods Market. Then you can add the calcium powder to food or beverages.

There are several important things to remember about calcium supplements. First, you should always purchase calcium with magnesium because the magnesium helps the body absorb the calcium. In addition, many calcium products have vitamin D, which is also important for absorption. Purchase the clear, tasteless forms. Take calcium twice a day, preferably in the morning and at night. Note that the body can only handle a limited amount of calcium at a time. If you ingest too much at one time, the body will flush out the excess. Finally, calcium supplements work best when they are taken with food.

Protein

By removing casein from the diet, a fair amount of protein disappears, too. Don't worry about that. Protein is protein, and it can be obtained in many other foods.

Protein is vital for cellular growth and repair. Protein helps in rebuilding muscles and generating new skin tissue. Another important function of protein is enzyme production. Enzymes break down food for digestion and have other functions in metabolic pathways. The U.S. recommended daily allowance of protein for children ages one to three is 13 grams. Children ages four to eight years old should have 19 grams every day. Children ages nine to thirteen should have 34 grams. At ages fourteen to eighteen, boys should have 52 grams and girls 46 grams every day. Protein can be found in meats, poultry, fish, beans, legumes, nuts, nut butters, rice, some bread, a few vegetables, and eggs. If soy is not a problem, many items that contain soy are loaded with protein, including soy milk.

Here is a list of items that contain protein and the amount of protein that each contains. The amounts may vary, based on how the foods are prepared.
- Egg, one, has 6 grams of protein.
- Fish*, 6 ounces, has 42 grams of protein.
- Crab*, 6 ounces, has 38 grams of protein.
- Shrimp*, 6 ounces, has 34 grams of protein.
- Beef, 6 ounces, has 38 grams of protein.
- Chicken, 6 ounces, has 42 grams of protein.
- Pork, 6 ounces, has 30 grams of protein.

- Kidney beans, one-half cup, have 8 grams of protein.
- Almonds, 1 ounce, have 6 grams of protein.
- Peanuts, 1 ounce, have 6 grams of protein.
- Brazil nuts, 1 ounce, have 6 grams of protein.
- Cashews, 1 ounce, have 6 grams of protein.
- Hazelnuts, 1 ounce, have 6 grams of protein.
- Pecans, 1 ounce, have 2 grams of protein.
- Pumpkin seeds, 2 ounces, have 19 grams of protein.
- Sunflower seeds, 2 ounces, have 6 grams of protein.
- Flax seeds, 2 ounces, have 8 grams of protein.
- Soybeans, 1 cup, have 22 grams of protein. (Make sure soy is tolerated.)
- Tofu, 5 ounces, has 10 grams of protein. (Make sure soy is tolerated.)
- Rice, 1 cup, has 3–7 grams of protein, depending on type of rice.
- Gluten-free grains, 1 cup, have 3–7 grams of protein, depending on type.
- Sweet corn, one cob, has 5 grams of protein.
- White beans, 1 cup, have 19 grams of protein.
- Lentils, 1 cup, have 18 grams of protein.
- Refried beans, 1 cup, have 14 grams of protein.
- Chickpeas or garbanzo beans, 1 cup, have 12 grams of protein.
- Lima beans, 1 cup, have 12 grams of protein.
- Navy beans, 1 cup, have 14 grams of protein.
- Peas, 1 cup, have 7 grams of protein.
- Potato, baked, one, has 5–7 grams of protein.
- Sweet potato, 1 cup, has 3 grams of protein.
- Avocado, one, has 4 grams of protein.
- Broccoli, 1 cup, has 3 grams of protein.
- Spinach, 1 cup, has 2 grams of protein.
- Bread, 1 slice, has 2–3 grams of protein.
- Peanut butter, 2 tablespoons, has 8 grams of protein.
- Cashew butter, 2 tablespoons, has 6 grams of protein.
- Sunflower butter, 2 tablespoons, has 6 grams of protein.
- Almond butter, 2 tablespoons, has 6 grams of protein.

*Beware of mercury levels in seafood and fish.

Fiber

You might feel that, because your child has stopped eating the usual grains, he or she will be missing out on fiber. This is untrue. Gluten-free grains have plenty of fiber.

Fruits and vegetables also have a decent amount of fiber. Of course, they are naturally GFCF. Be aware, though, that many fruits can cause yeast build-up in the intestines. Some fruits have phenols, while others have salicylates. Because of your child's reaction to these substances, you may need to avoid some fruits. Don't give your child fruit until you have read about phenols and salicylates in Chapter 13.

Fiber has several important roles in the body. Fiber intake helps lower cholesterol and assists with waste elimination. Fiber is also important to weight management and blood sugar control. Some incidences of cancer can be reduced with appropriate fiber consumption. There are several theories on how much fiber a child needs every day. Some sources state that a child should have their age plus 5 grams of fiber. For example, a two-year-old needs 7 grams; a ten-year-old needs 15 grams, and so on. However, the American Dietetic Association's website (http://www.eatright.org) recommends 19 grams of fiber for ages one to three, and 25 grams for ages four to six. For ages nine to thirteen, boys need 31 grams daily, and girls need 26 grams. Many other resources say this level is very high and difficult to attain. Use your own judgment, and seek advice from your doctor.

A great way to get fiber while on a GFCF Diet is by eating some of the following foods.
- Pear, 1 medium, has 5 grams of fiber.
- Figs, dried, 2 medium, have 4 grams of fiber.
- Blueberries, 1 cup, have 4 grams of fiber.
- Apricots, dried, 10 halves, have 3 grams of fiber.
- Orange, 1 medium, has 3 grams of fiber.

- Strawberries, 1 cup, have 3 grams of fiber.
- Raspberries, 1 cup, have 10 grams of fiber.
- Banana, one, has 3 grams of fiber.
- Lentils, 1 cup, have 15 grams of fiber.
- Black beans, 1 cup, have 15 grams of fiber.
- Lima beans, 1 cup, have 13 grams of fiber.
- Peas, 1 cup, have 9 grams of fiber.
- Corn, 1 cup, has 4 grams of fiber.
- Corn, 1 cob, has 5 grams of fiber.
- Spinach, cooked, 1/2 cup, has 7 grams of fiber.
- Yam, 1 medium, has 7 grams of fiber.
- Potato, 1 small, has 5 grams of fiber.
- Popcorn, 3 cups, has 4 grams of fiber.
- Carrot, 1 medium, has 2 grams of fiber.
- Peanuts, 1 ounce, have 3 grams of fiber.
- Brown rice bread, 1 slice, has 2 grams of fiber.
- Brown rice pasta, 2 ounces, has 2 grams of fiber.

Always choose brown rice over white rice for more fiber. Before cooking, one half-cup of brown rice has 6 grams of fiber, while the same amount of white rice only has 2 grams. Many of the bean flours in Bette Hagman's recipes have a high level of fiber.

Great Food Preparation Tips

People following the GFCF Diet have come up with fantastic tips for purchasing and preparing these foods. I've provided some of the best tips for you here.

Replace Milk with Club Soda

Use club soda in pancake and waffle mixes to replace the milk. The soda makes the pancakes and waffles much fluffier and tastier. Think about hiding some flaxseed or shredded vegetables in your recipes to make them even healthier. Hansen Beverage Company makes a good, natural club soda.

The Best Bread Maker

Many people with celiac disease say the best bread maker is Zojirushi Corporation's Home Bakery machine. The bread maker has two paddles that help with GF mixes and ingredients. The company includes GF recipes with the product guide. The bread machine makes a 1.5- to 2-pound loaf that looks just like a typical loaf of bread. You may use mixes, too. Gluten Evolution's Breads from Anna mixes (http://www. glutenevolution.com) come highly recommended. Ingredients are listed on the company's website. Some of the mixes are GFCF, and some are even GFCFSF.

Xanthan Gum

One ingredient that is a must for baking with gluten-free flours is xanthan gum. You can purchase a bag of it from Bob's Red Mill or a small jar from several different manufacturers at a variety of stores. You will only need a small amount for most recipes, so the gum should last you a long time. Xanthan gum helps add elasticity to GF breads, cakes, and cookies, something that GF flours are missing.

Decorating Desserts

When you are decorating cookies and cakes, you will need to use natural, GFCF dyes and sprinkles. You can order them online from the websites listed here, or you can find them in health-food stores or specialty stores.

- India Tree Gourmet Spices and Specialties (http://www.indiatree. com/products/decorative/index.html)
- Nature's Flavors (http://www.naturesflavors.com/default. php?cPath=72)

- Edward & Sons Trading Company (http://edwardandsons.com/Zero_Gluten_Products.html)
- You can even make your own GFCF dyes and sprinkles with recipes found at the following website:
  - Lakewinds (http://www.lakewinds.com/store/Natural-Egg-Dye-Recipes-W4698C18760.aspx)
  - In the spring, Whole Foods and other companies usually post recipes for how to make natural dyes; search online for "natural dye recipes."

Pet Foods

Pet foods often have gluten in them, and they also can contain casein. Read the labels. Call the companies. Children can easily pick up pet food or perhaps be licked by a pet that just ate some. You can never be too careful.

Candy

Kids love candy and, as much as we want to keep candy away from them, sometimes we do not want them to feel left out. An occasional treat is okay. First, make sure the candy label does not list artificial dyes or preservatives among the ingredients. Next, check to see if it is GFCF. Here are a few brands of acceptable candy, most of which are available at Whole Foods Market, at health-food stores, and online. (Websites for some additional chocolate companies are listed in Chapter 3.)

- College Farm Organic lollipops and hard candy, http://www.collegefarmorganic.com or 1-800-367-2441
- Yummy Earth Organic lollipops, http://www.yummyearth.com or 1-201.857-8489
- Tropical Source chocolate bars, http://www.sunspire.com or 1-800-434-4246

- Jelly Belly (only some are dye free and GFCF), http://www.jellybelly.com or 1-800-522-3267
- Edward & Sons Organic Gummi Bears (three varieties), Black Licorice Bears, and Gummi Feet, http://edwardandsons.com/let_do_organic.html or 1-805-684-8500
- Giambri's Quality Sweets, http://www.giambriscandy.com or 1-856-783-1099

You can make your own candy by buying plastic molds from stores such as Michaels, Jo-Ann's, or a local craft shop. Here are simple instructions to get you started.

Use Tropical Source bars or GFCF chocolate chips and plastic molds. Put the chocolate and a small amount of cooking oil in a glass container. Heat the mixture in the microwave oven for a few seconds, just until the chocolate melts. Stir until smooth.

Pour the mixture into the molds. Put them immediately in the freezer and wait ten to fifteen minutes. When the bottom of the mold starts to turn white, the candy is ready to come out. Turn the molds over, and you have cute, little chocolate shapes.

You also can get lollipop sticks and turn your molded shapes into lollipops. Before you put the mold in the freezer, twirl the sticks into the chocolate so that the end of each stick is covered.

GF Flours

Buy your GF flours in bulk at Asian markets. Combine them into flour mixes, as listed in Chapter 5, and keep them in the pantry or freezer (as shown in the storage chart, also in Chapter 5). This way, whenever you are ready to bake, especially around holiday times, you will have already done most of the hard work.

Smoothies

Get a smoothie maker. (A blender can work, too.) You can use GF rice milk, soy milk (if tolerated), coconut milk, almond milk, hemp milk, or DariFree. Another option is to add juices, your choice of frozen fruits (only 100 percent fruit), and 100 percent natural sorbet. (Häagen-Dazs, Sharon's Sorbet, Dreyer's-Edy's, Ciao Bella, and Ben & Jerry's are all good, natural brands.) Whirl up some healthy concoctions. Add powdered calcium or other supplements, if desired.

Popsicles

Make your own popsicles. Use 100 percent juice or a natural, homemade smoothie mixture. Freeze the liquid in molds for a healthy summer treat.

Vacationing

Before you leave on vacation, print out a list of all of the markets you may pass that carry GFCF foods, as well as those in the town where you will be staying. If a map is not included, go to Mapquest (http://www.mapquest.com) and print one out. First, try the main stores, if they will be near you: Whole Foods Market and Trader Joe's. Next, go to http://www.yellowpages.com (or http://www.numberway.com for international phone numbers) and look up "grocers" or "health foods." Enter the location of the area you will be visiting to obtain a list of the stores. You might even want to keep a list of the stores in your car. You can find a list of organic food stores in the United States at the Organic Consumers Association (http://www.organicconsumers.org/foodcoops.htm).

Chapter 7

⫸ How to Read Labels ⫷

Reading labels in stores can be very labor intensive. Since the U.S. Food Allergen Labeling and Consumer Protection Act became law, reading a label on a food product has become much easier. However, some questionable ingredients on labels still may not be explained fully. Labels for non-food products can also be hard to interpret. Since gluten is not listed as one of the top eight allergens (only wheat is), barley, rye, spelt, and other gluten grains do not have to be mentioned on the label.

Picking organic or 100 percent natural foods are your best bets. Be careful of the words "natural," or "healthy," because food companies use these misleading terms to try to entice consumers to purchase their products. The label must state that a product is organic or 100 percent natural for it to be free of chemicals and preservatives.

When I shop at my healthy-option stores I can pick up a can of pineapple and read just "pineapple and water" on the label. When I pick up a jar of peanut butter, the label reads, "peanuts and salt." It is very refreshing to understand what foods' ingredients are and to know that they are normal, healthy, and edible.

But many people don't shop at health-food stores, because they do not live near them or other healthier stores. When I was writing this chapter,

I ventured out to a traditional grocery store for the first time in a long time. I was shocked as I went from aisle to aisle, picking up one food product after another, at how many packages had odd ingredients and unexplained words listed. If you must shop at a traditional food store, or even if you can shop at a health-food store, this chapter should help you make the best food choices for your family.

Reading for Gluten or Casein Ingredients

Here is a list of some words that you should know, because they could mean the presence of gluten or casein in the foods you buy. If you are in doubt, contact the company's customer service departments to verify. If you see these following ingredients listed, you should not consume the product because it is not GFCF. The items marked with an asterisk could be from corn or another GF grain. If so, these items would be fine to consume on the GFCF Diet. But be aware that these items frequently are manufactured from gluten and thus should be avoided. They could also contain preservatives.

WORDS MEANING GLUTEN

- Wheat
- Flour (of course, not GF types of flour)
- Oats (from contamination)
- Barley
- Rye
- Spelt
- Malt
- Triticum
- Durum
- Bulgur
- Fu
- Kamut

- Couscous
- Semolina
- Soy sauce (it contains wheat)
- Hydrolyzed vegetable protein (HVP)*
- Hydrolyzed plant protein (HPP)*
- Modified food starch*
- Natural flavoring*
- Vinegar* (If distilled, it is GF, as this process removes the gluten.)

WORDS MEANING CASEIN

- Milk
- Dairy
- Whey
- Curds
- Caseinate
- Cream
- Butter
- Lactose
- Margarine **
- Cheese **
- Yogurt **
- Pudding **
- Ice cream **
- Caramel **
- Lactic Acid Starter Culture **

Items marked with ** in the list above could be derived from soy but considered GFCF, if no other gluten or casein is found in the product. If you are avoiding soy, you will need to avoid these foods. Some of these options are derived from rice and thus may be GFCF.

Ingredient Label Examples

Over time, you will become an expert at label reading. But to start, the best way to learn is to work with some examples. Here are some ingredient labels and explanations on how to decipher whether the product is GFCF. I will mention any ingredients that could possibly be gluten or casein, so you know what to look out for. If in doubt, you can call the company.

Item 1. Nature Valley Snack Bar

almonds, peanuts, sunflower seeds, sugar, corn syrup, salt

Nothing here indicates that the bar has gluten, casein, or soy in it.

Item 2. Glutino Gluten Free Apple & Cinnamon Cereal

corn flour, corn starch, cane juice, dried apples, canola oil, d-alpha to-copheryl, acetate and d-alpha tocopherol (vitamin E), baking powder, apple and cinnamon flavor, honey, salt
may contain traces of tree nuts, sesame, soy, and milk.

This package has been marked gluten free by a reliable company that makes GF foods. Some people may have issues with traces of milk, while others will not. Baking powder can have gluten in it, too, but the cereal manufacturer is a GF company, so you know you are safe. Tocopherol is just another name for vitamin E, sometimes found containing soy. However, this label says the product may contain just traces, not that it does contain soy. Acetate is a form of vitamin E.

Item 3. MimicCreme, Sweetened

purified water, sugar, almonds, cashews, maltodextrin, tapioca starch, guar gum, salt, bicarbonate soda

This product is labeled gluten free, nondairy (pareve), and soy free. The unsweetened formula of MimicCreme has no sugar, no maltodextrin, and no guar gum. It also uses rice starch instead of tapioca starch. The sweetened, sugar-free formula uses erythritol, a 100 percent natural sugar substitute. The sugar-free formula also uses tapioca starch and guar gum. These two formulas are GFCFSF.

Maltodextrin is a carbohydrate usually derived from rice, corn, or potato starch. It is not derived from malt or barley, so it is GFCF. (Remember, the package says this product is GFCFSF). The bicarbonate soda (baking soda) is also GF in this food. You can be sure of this because the label says GF. All three formulas also are labeled as pareve and vegan, which means they cannot have any milk derivatives. So this product is GFCFSF. MimicCreme is a substitute for whipping cream. It can be used to make ice cream, creamy desserts, "creamed" soup, creamy sauces, and anything that requires regular cream.

Item 4. FreeZees Fudgee Fudge

pureed cashew, organic agave syrup (a low glycemic index ingredient), amaranth, & quinoa, inulin (a probiotic ingredient from chicory), isolated soy protein, fudge/carob flavor, guar & xanthan gum, soy lecithin & sea salt

The label states the product is vegan, so you know it is casein free. Nothing indicates it has gluten in it. There is soy in the product, as stated on the label.

Item 5. Glutino Corn Bread

---

water, corn starch, tapioca starch, safflower oil, evaporated cane juice, dried egg whites, salt, guar gum, glucono-delta-lactone, yeast*, pectic, sodium bicarbonate, sodium alginate, modified vegetable cellulose, thiamine, niacin, vitamin b6, riboflavin, iron, calcium
*Order may vary.
May contain traces of soy.

The package states that the corn bread is gluten free, wheat free, milk free, and casein free, so it is GFCF. The label also indicates it is free of trans-fatty acids and cholesterol, and has neither refined sugar nor hydrogenated oils. After contacting the company, I found out about the other odd ingredients. Glucono-delta-lactone is a food additive used as a leavening agent. Sodium alginate is the sodium salt of alginic acid, which is used in the food industry to increase viscosity and act as an emulsifier. Modified vegetable cellulose is used as a thickening agent.

Item 6. Wolfgang Puck Organic Chicken with White and Wild Rice Soup

---

organic chicken stock (water, chicken meat and natural juices, salt, cane sugar, maltodextrin, natural flavor, dried onion, potato starch, dried garlic turmeric and spice extractives), organic carrots, organic cooked chicken meat, organic white rice, organic potato starch, organic wild rice, contains 2% or less of the following: organic onions, organic celery, organic chicken fat, organic spice, organic paprika, organic turmeric

---

The label does not say gluten free, so you do not know if the malto-dextrin and natural flavors are from gluten or not. Nothing looks like casein here, but without asking the company, you do not know if the soup is GFCF. By going to Wolfgang Puck's website and looking under FAQs (http://wolfgangpucksoup.com/faq.shtml#q3), you will find the answers to these questions. The website states: "Currently, the Wolfgang Puck Soup varieties that *do not* contain gluten are: Roast Chicken w/Wild Rice, Hearty Lentil & Vegetables, Chicken Tortilla, Roast Chicken w/Rice & Rosemary (formerly Grilled Chicken w/ Rice), Organic Thick Hearty Lentil & Vegetables, Organic Chicken w/White & Wild Rice, Organic Creamy Butternut Squash, Organic Tortilla, Organic Spicy Bean, Organic French Onion, and Organic Split Pea. *You should check the labels of each individual variety because we occasionally make improvements by changing ingredients.* The All Natural Free Range Roasted Chicken Stock, as well as the Organic Beef Broth, Organic Chicken Broth, and the Organic Vegetable Broth are also gluten free.

"Four of our ingredients contain the milk protein, casein. These ingredients are: butter, heavy cream, parmesan cheese, and cream flavor. The following Wolfgang Puck Soup varieties *do not* contain these ingredients and could be considered casein free: Chicken & Egg Noodles, Hearty Lentil & Vegetables, Hearty Vegetable Beef, Roast Chicken w/Vegetables, Old Fashion Beef Barley, Roast Chicken w/Wild Rice, Roasted Chicken w/White Wine & Fine Herbs, Roasted Chicken w/ Egg Noodles & Rosemary, Savory Pot Roast w/Vegetables, Chicken Tortilla, Roast Chicken w/Rice & Rosemary (formerly Grilled Chicken w/Rice), Organic Thick Hearty Lentil & Vegetables, Organic Tortilla, Organic Spicy Bean, Organic Chicken w/White & Wild Rice, and Organic Chicken w/Egg Noodles. All of our stocks and broths are casein free."

Item 7. Newman's Own Dressing, Light Raspberry and Walnut

> *water, sugar, vegetable oil, (soybean and/or canola) oil, red wine vinegar, corn syrup solids, raspberry, walnuts, salt, natural flavors, orange juice concentrate, onion, xanthan gum, spices, natural elderberry extract and annatto (for color)*

Natural flavors and red wine vinegar are two ingredients to investigate further to see if they contain gluten. Distilled vinegar is GF, because any gluten grains are removed during the distillation process. But be careful about vinegar that is not marked "distilled." Usually it will still be GF. Malt vinegar absolutely has gluten in it and must be avoided. Annatto is a natural-colored pulp surrounding the seeds of a tree called *Bixa orellana*, which grows in the tropical regions of the Americas. Annatto is added to many foods to achieve a yellow-orange coloring and is GFCF.

Newman's Own's website has a chart showing some allergens, including gluten and milk, that may be in the company's products (http://newmansown.com/faqs.cfm#q6). This chart states that there is no milk and no gluten in this product. Consult this list for other products because some Newman's Own dressings contain milk and gluten. No milk means no casein for this product.

Item 8. 365 Brand Semi-sweet Chocolate Chips

> *sugar, chocolate liquor, cocoa butter, soy lecithin (emulsifier), vanilla extract*

Vanilla extract could be made with alcohol, which could contain gluten. Whole Foods Market, this product's manufacturer, has verified it being GFCF, so no gluten was used in the vanilla extract. However, the chocolate chips do contain soy. Cocoa butter is from chocolate and is not a dairy product.

Item 9. Canned Tomatoes

tomatoes, tomato juice, high fructose corn syrup, salt, dehydrated onion, dehydrated celery, dehydrated bell pepper, calcium chloride, citric acid, oregano, basil, natural flavoring

The only thing questionable could be the natural flavoring. HFCS is not a great ingredient, in terms of basic health, but it is gluten free and casein free. Calcium chloride is used as a form of salt to preserve foods.

Item 10. Clams

clams in their natural juices, water, salt, sugar, sodium tripolyphosphate (to retain natural juices), calcium disodium EDTA (to protect color)

Sodium tripolyphosphate is a crystalline salt used to preserve foods, thus it is a preservative. Calcium disodium EDTA is a synthetic compound and stabilizer in food supplements. It is used as a preservative. Avoid!

Item 11. 365 Brand Cherry Vanilla Crème Soda

filtered carbonated water, pure cane sugar, natural cherry vanilla flavor and citric acid

There is no cream or crème in this soda; that is merely the name of the soda. The can states that there are no artificial colors, no artificial flavors, no preservatives, and no caffeine, and that the product is all natural.

Chapter 8

⋙ Eating Out, Vacationing, ⋘ and Hospital Visits

What about eating out?

Eating out can be complicated, but it is far from impossible. With more and more restaurant personnel being trained about allergies and intolerances, you will find more people understanding what cross-contamination means (more on this is in Chapter 6) and the importance of keeping foods separate.

With one in 133 people being diagnosed with celiac disease (an intolerance to gluten that seriously impacts the intestinal tract), more and more restaurants are introducing gluten-free menu items. *Eating out is still very risky.* The more precautions you take, the better. Dealing with preservatives outside of your home is much more difficult to manage. When you are ordering, make sure that the staff understands that your food must also be casein free and dye free. Often, the best bet is asking the manager to come to your table. He or she should go the extra mile to assure that your food is safe. You might suggest cooking some of the foods on foil to avoid cross-contamination from the grill.

Here are some special ways to order food, after you make sure it is free of intolerances:

- Order a 100 percent meat burger or chicken breast wrapped in lettuce—or just plain, no bun. (Make sure there is no coating, nor anything else added to the food that is not GFCF.)
- Order a plain baked potato or corn on the cob, no butter.
- Order raw or steamed vegetables, no butter, or fruit.
- Ask to read labels of sauces, spices, or other toppings.
- Ask whether the oil used for french fries is used for anything but plain potatoes. Nothing that has wheat, wheat coating, other gluten forms, or dairy products can be fried in the same oil, or the fries will become contaminated. Ask if the fries are cooked in a dedicated fryer where nothing else can fall in or come in contact with the french fries. Explain this very carefully, because many people will not understand what you mean.

Here are some restaurants in the United States that provide GF menus or items. Be aware that most of these listings are only for gluten-free places. You will have to contact the restaurant to see if they offer casein-free foods and can accommodate other allergens or intolerances that you must avoid. Check the restaurant's website or call first. Print out the menu, and bring it in with you. Many of these restaurants are nationwide in the United States, but some are only in several states or specific regions. (Some restaurants outside the United States are posted below the U.S. list, with many more listed in the Resources section at the end of this book.)

Austin Grill (http://www.austingrill.com)
Biaggi's (http://www.biaggis.com/restaurants.htm)
Bonefish Grill (http://www.bonefishgrill.com)
Bugaboo Creek Steak House (http://www.bugaboocreek.com)
Burger King (http://www.bk.com)
Cameron Mitchell restaurants (http://www.cameronmitchell.com/restaurants/index.cfm)
Carino's (http://www.carinos.com/menu/gluten-free.aspx)

Carrabba's Italian Grill (http://www.carrabbas.com/menu.asp)

Charlie Brown's Steakhouse (http://www.charliebrowns.com/menu.shtml)

Cheeseburger in Paradise (http://www.cheeseburgerinparadise.com/gluten-free-menu.asp)

Chick-fil-a (http://www.chick-fil-a.com/gluten.asp)

Chili's Grill and Bar (http://www.chilis.com)

Claim Jumper (http://www.claimjumper.com/hypertext/menu_diet_gluten.htm)

Don Pablo's (http://www.donpablos.com)

Firebirds Wood Fired Grill (http://www.firebirdsrockymountaingrill.com)

Fresh City (http://www.freshcity.com/fastLink_glutenfree.html)

First Watch (http://www.firstwatch.com/glutenfree.htm)

Kona Grill (http://www.konagrill.com/menu.php?cid=15)

Legal Sea Foods (http://www.legalseafoods.com/)

O'Charley's (http://www.ocharleys.com/allergen/)

The Old Spaghetti Factory (http://www.osf.com)

On the Border (http://www.ontheborder.com)

Outback Steakhouse (http://www.outback.com)

Pei Wei Asian Diner (http://www.peiwei.com)

P.F. Chang's China Bistro (http://www.pfchangs.com)

Pizza Fusion (http://www.pizzafusion.com/menu/)

Rafferty's Restaurant & Bar (http://www.raffertys.com)

Red Robin (http://redrobin.com); go to FAQs; see allergens.

Romano's Macaroni Grill (http://www.macaronigrill.com)

Rubio's Fresh Mexican Grill (http://www.rubios.com)

Taco Del Mar (http://www.tacodelmar.com/food/gluten.html)

Ted's Montana Grill (http://tedsmontanagrill.com/nutrition_gluten_free.html)

Uno Chicago Grill (http://www.unos.com/kiosk/nutritionUnos.html)

Wendy's (http://www.wendys.com)

Wildfire (http://www.wildfirerestaurant.com/second_level/menu/celiac.htm)

Winger's Grill & Bar (http://wingers.info/glutenmenu.html)

Z'Teja's Southwestern Grill (http://www.ztejas.com)

For dairy-free restaurant options, go to GoDairyFree.org (http://www.godairyfree.org/Table/Dining-Out/Suggested-Restaurants). Make sure your choices are also gluten free.

Many people on the GFCF Diet long for mall-style hot pretzels. Look no further than Noah's Pretzels (http://www.noahspretzels.com), which also are soy free. The company opened up in 2007 in the Washington, DC, area but will ship baked, ready-to-heat pretzels to your door. Two dads started this company. One of them has a son, Noah, who has ASD. They donate some of their profits to autism-related causes. Their pretzels are even sold at the Washington Nationals stadium and the Verizon Center.

Bakeries serving GF and some GFCF breads and sweets are cropping up all over the place. Here are some to check out. Many of them will ship their items all over the United States.

New Cascadia Traditional (http://www.newcascadiatraditional.com)

Cute as Cake (http://www.cuteascake.com)

Gluuteny Bakery (http://www.gluuteny.com)

Lori Bakes Gluten Free (http://loribake.startlogic.com/bakeryandcafe.htm)

Mariposa Baking Company (http://www.mariposabaking.com)

The Sensitive Baker (http://store.thesensitivebaker.com)

Green Cupcakes & More (http://www.greencupcakes.com)

If you want GFCF prepared entrees to heat up, plus side dishes and baked goods, all delivered to your home or an alternative site with an oven, contact GF Meals (http://www.gfmeals.com). The company delivers all over the United States.

Here are some sources of international restaurants offering GF or GFCF meals. For more restaurant listings, see international sites listed in the Resources section at the end of this book.

United States:

Gluten-Free Restaurant Awareness Program (http://www.glutenfreerestaurants.org)

Gluten Free Registry (http://www.glutenfreeregistry.com)
Gluten-Free Globe (http://www.glutenfreeglobe.com/destinations.
php)
Canada:
Celiac Canada (http://www.penny.ca/Travel.htm)
Australia and New Zealand: (http://members.ozemail.com.
au/~coeliac/dine.html)
United Kingdom:
Gluten-Free Places (http://glutenfreeplaces.com)
Around the world (only some countries are listed):
Gluten-free on the go (http://www.gluten-free-onthego.com)
GlutenFree Passport (http://www.glutenfreepassport.com)
CeliacHandbook.com (http://www.celiachandbook.com/
restaurant-guide.html)

For restaurants not listed here, you usually will need to ask for the manager to arrange for your food to be GFCF. Explain in detail what GFCF means and that the food for you and your child cannot contain any gluten or casein—or even come in contact with them via utensils, pans, or the grill. If you explain it like a serious allergy, you often get treated more seriously. You can obtain cards to keep in your wallet that give information about the diet and that you can present to your server or to the manager. You can order them from:

- *Living Without* magazine (http://www.livingwithout.com/dining-cards.html),
- DietaryCard.com (http://www.dietarycard.com), available in nineteen languages,
- Select Wisely (http://www.selectwisely.com), in more than forty languages, or
- CeliacTravel.com (http://www.celiactravel.com/restaurant-cards.html), in forty-two languages.

TRUE STORIES IN THE GF AND GFCF WORLD

Here are a few interesting and true on-the-road conversations showing how clueless people can be regarding ingredients in food and other products. I am sure you will find many stories of your own in your quest to educate the public about GFCF.

Mom: My son cannot eat the bun. He is allergic to wheat!
Waiter: Our buns are white, not wheat.
Mom: All bread found in restaurants, whether white or wheat, is made from the wheat plant, thus white bread *is wheat*.
Waiter: Oh!

Mom: My son needs a bunless burger.
Cashier: We don't have any bunless burgers.
Mom: I mean a burger without the bun.
Cashier: Oh! Sure, we can do that.

Customer at restaurant: I can't eat wheat, so no toast, please.
Waitress: Do you want bread instead?
Customer at restaurant: No! No bread, no toast. Toast is bread that has been in a toaster. It contains wheat. Toast is bread.
Waitress: Okay, sure, got it.

Women in a hotel: You don't stick to your special diet on vacations, do you?
Woman with celiac disease: Of course I do; I have no choice. I can't be chained to my hotel room.

Customer: I can't have anything with wheat—no rolls, no wheat, no bread.
Waitress: Our stuff is not made from wheat. It's made from flour.
Customer: Flour is made from wheat. Do you remember the story of the little red hen?

> Customer: I would like my burger prepared without a bun. I can't have wheat, so I can't have the hamburger bun.
>
> Waitress: *(Getting very excited)* Hold on! I can help you! *(She comes running back and holds up a package of hot dog buns.)* If you're allergic to hamburger buns, I can cut the meat to fit in the hot dog bun for you!
>
> Sadly, those and many other similar stories are not rare. Explaining what you need as meticulously as possible will help the wait staff to understand you better. Again, eating away from home can be very risky.

What about vacationing?

While eating out or vacationing, you can always pack your own food in a cooler to avoid problems. Restaurants and theme parks are not allowed to prohibit this, as long as you explain that you need the food because of strict dietary restrictions. A note from your doctor is not a bad idea, just in case the park staff has concerns about you bringing your own food. Guest Relations might need to approve of the foods being brought into the park or site.

You can purchase a backpack with a built-in cooler to carry around your food. Here are a few that are available online:

- Overstock.com (http://www.overstock.com/Sports-Toys/Deluxe-Backpack-Cooler/2064058/product.html?cid=25608&fp=F)
- Keep Your Cooler.com (http://www.keepyourcooler.com/backpack-coolers.html)
- BeverageFactory.com (http://www.beveragefactory.com/wine/picnic/backpack.shtml)
- BagKing.com (http://www.bagking.com/Merchant2/merchant.mvc?Screen=CTGY&Category_Code=04-2-2)
- eBags.com (http://www.ebags.com/picnic_time/zuma/product_detail/index.cfm?modelid=85409)

Renting a locker at an amusement park is a good idea so you are not stuck carrying your backpack or cooler with you all day. Most lockers have all-day open-and-close privileges for a set fee. That means you can visit your locker throughout the day without paying each time you open it.

If you are on vacation in the United States and need to keep your special foods cold in the hotel room, have a refrigerator delivered to your room. You should *never* pay for one to be brought to your room and kept there during your stay. Explain to the reservation operator or hotel clerk ahead of time that your child or you have special needs and require special foods. It is illegal under the Americans with Disabilities Act of 1990 for any hotel to charge you for accommodations needed by those with disabilities. If hotel staff fight you on this, mention the law and you will get your refrigerator free. In other countries, you will have to ask if they can accommodate your needs.

The best places to vacation while on a GFCF Diet are the Disney parks. They are very understanding about special dietary needs. Call ahead of time to alert them that you will be arriving at a certain time and date. If you are booking a character meal, tell them you will need a GFCF and dye-free meal.

Disney restaurants are amazing at preparing special dishes. The chef will come to your table and write down, in detail, exactly what he or she can do to give you the best dining experience. The food will arrive separately at your table. The restaurants have separate grills, pans, and waffle irons—and they will go the extra mile or kilometer to keep food safe from cross-contamination.

Disney Dining does not have toll-free numbers. For Walt Disney World, Florida, call: 1-407-WDW-DINE. For Disneyland-California Adventure, California, call: 1-714-781-DINE. Disney also can send you a list in advance of all of the concessions, restaurants, and food locations in the park that have GFCF foods.

Here are some other great vacation options:

- Disneyland Paris has a wonderful PDF file written by a dietician who discusses many allergy-free options within the park. The park's website (http://www.disneylandparis.com/index2.jsp?c=0#) is available in many different languages. Just click on the flag or the language on the list that represents the one that you need. For the English version of the file on allergy-free options, download http://www.disneylandparis.co.uk/UK/EN/Neutral/Images/food_allergies_uk.pdf.
- Many of the park's allergy-free meals are available for all patrons, but some require advance notice and reservations. Call +33 (0) 1 60 30 40 50 and discuss your dietary needs with the reservationist. Make sure that you call in plenty of time before your arrival date.
- For Hong Kong Disneyland to handle special diets, you will need to contact park staff before your visit and explain your family's dietary needs. You can reach them in Hong Kong at (852) 3510 3388.
- Holiday World & Splashin' Safari in Santa Claus, Indiana, offers many foods that are free of all of the eight top allergens and also GF (http://www.holidayworld.com/food.html). The park's 500 food employees have received specialized training on food allergies.
- Legoland in San Diego, California, also makes excellent accommodations for special diets. Call at least seventy-two hours ahead of your visit to speak with the executive chef. He will adjust the menu to suit your needs. Your food will be kept separately until you arrive to ask for it. The staff will even get french fries from another park area with a dedicated fryer (just for fries) and bring the food to your table. Contact them at: http://www.legoland.com/park/Dining/dietaryconcerns.htm or 760-846-0876.
- For Legoland in Windsor, UK, to meet your dietary needs, contact the park at least twenty-four hours before your visit. Allow more time during popular seasons. To learn more, go to

http://www.legoland.co.uk/planyourvisit/faq.htm#dietary and click on "Dietary Requirements."

- Legoland in Billund, Denmark, does not specify any dietary information on the park's website (http://www.legoland.dk). Contact them to ask for assistance.
- Legoland in Günzburg, Germany, also does not specify dietary information on its website (http://www.legoland.de/?lc=en). Contact them to ask for assistance.
- For other theme parks, contact the dining department or guest relations and ask for the head chef to discuss how they can accommodate your or your child's special dietary needs.

Another wonderful option for those with special dietary needs is a vacation on a cruise ship. You must inform the special needs department at least ninety days prior to sailing, although even earlier is better. Most cruise lines go above and beyond to accommodate guests with special diets. You will probably be instructed to consult with the maître d', not the waiter, upon entering the dining room for each meal. People on restricted diets, specifically gluten free, have enjoyed and have been happily accommodated by these cruise lines: Celebrity, Carnival, Royal Caribbean, and Princess.

For assistance with gluten-free traveling, check out Bob and Ruth's Gluten-Free Dining & Traveling Club website (http://www.bobandruths.com). Inform them that you need to be casein free, too.

What about hospital stays?

If you or your child has to spend time in the hospital, you will need to ask about the food and medications that will be provided. Ask the hospital personnel to give you or your child (the patient) an allergy bracelet stating everything that he or she must not consume. You might want to bring in meals or having someone bring them for you, if the hospital staff does not seem to understand your requests or comply with them, or both.

The best bet might be for your doctor to have a dietician visit to walk you through meal planning. The dietician can provide you with GFCF menus and adjust them according to your needs. The food service personnel will be alerted to the requirements of your or your child's dietary requests.

Chapter 9

❧ The GFCF Diet in Action: ❧ Questions and Answers

As you begin the diet, you will certainly have many questions. Below are a few commonly asked questions and the answers.

General Questions

Q. What are some ideas for packing school lunches?

A. Get a metal-lined thermos. (Some people prefer not to use anything metal; see the next question for more detail.) Mark the thermos "GFCF," so you know never to use it for foods that can contaminate.

Here's a way to keep food hot until lunch. First, wash out the thermos and let it dry. Fill a microwavable glass cup with water, and put it in the microwave. Heat for about two minutes. Then pour the water into the thermos and let it sit. Meanwhile, put GFCF foods—such as soup, chicken, or pasta and sauce—into a microwavable glass container and heat it in the microwave for two minutes. When it is done, pour the hot water out of the thermos and fill it with the food. This should stay hot for several hours.

Try leftover meals from the night before: meat loaf, chicken and rice, casseroles, cut-up hot dogs and BBQ sauce, or ground meat sauce. Be creative. Always add a sauce because it helps keep the food warm in the thermos.

Another option for lunches are sandwiches. You can try peanut butter or other nut butters and jelly; nut butters and bananas (if phenols are not a problem); nut butters with any other interesting allowed fruits; or nitrite- and nitrate-free GFCF lunch meats. You can add rice cakes, pancakes, or waffles—or even use them as bread for your sandwich. Add snack bars, chips, nuts, fruit leathers, and fruits and veggies. For a change of pace, you can send cereal and a milk alternative. (Put the "milk" in a tightly sealed container.)

Q. Should I be worried about a metal container?

A. Some people might not want to use a metal thermos because of its aluminum content, which some believe can cause neurotoxic harm. That is your decision. You will be able to find plastic thermoses, but they do not keep foods warm for long.

Q. Do I have to shop at a health-food store to obtain all of these foods?

A. No, but shopping at Whole Foods Market, Trader Joe's, or a health-food store would make it a lot easier. The regular grocery store will have some GFCF foods. Many markets have specialty food sections where you may be able to locate GFCF products. However, you have to be very good at reading labels and making phone calls. Many people order GFCF foods online. Remember, many single-ingredient foods—such as meats, poultry, fruits, vegetables, eggs, and nuts—are GFCF as long as they are without additives.

Q. Do I have to get a Defeat Autism Now! doctor? Will any doctor be able to help us?

A. You do not need to find a doctor who has attended training sessions at Defeat Autism Now! conferences. You can use your regular pediatrician, but you most likely will have to bring him or her the research that you find. Many general doctors are not up on the latest information, and many will pooh-pooh it.

Bring in magazine articles, medical journal entries, and other data that you can print out online. Be strong; share results with your doctor. If you are not happy with the doctor, find a new one. Ask in support groups or via word of mouth for well-known, well-liked pediatricians who have the same philosophies as you.

You should be able to interview doctors without paying for an appointment. You'll want to find one with whom you feel comfortable and who will work with you, with an open mind, to help your child without always wanting to prescribe drugs. There are alternatives to drugs, and doctors should be open to these approaches.

Q. What are some of the great GFCF foods or places to eat at the Disney parks?

A. Make your reservations early. You can call up to six months in advance to book a table at the more popular restaurants. Contact Disney's chef several days before your visit to discuss GFCF foods. Also mention your special dietary needs when you make your reservation.

McDonald's hosted carts and a few restaurants in the parks have dedicated GFCF french fries. (McDonald's has received media attention for its fries perhaps not being GFCF, so verify before eating them.) Many restaurants will provide GFCF buns if you call ahead to order them. Many locations in the park can also provide rice pasta.

Main Street Ice Cream Parlour (located on Main Street) carries GFCF Rice Dream ice cream and Tofutti, which are not soy free. Many character breakfast places have GFCF waffles and pancakes. They can provide soy milk and orange juice in closed containers to avoid cross-contamination. All of the carts throughout the park carry frozen fruit bars that are GFCF and dye free. The turkey drumsticks sold in carts in several of the parks also are GFCF, although they may have preservatives.

Q. Can I start my teenager on the GFCF Diet?

A. Sure. Many people have had great success in starting the diet with teens. The process might be more challenging, but the success rate should be the same as for a younger child.

Q. Why is it that some lists do not mention oats as having gluten?

A. Oats by themselves do not contain gluten. But most oats are cross-contaminated with wheat while in the fields, so most lists state that oats are not GF. GF-guaranteed oats exist, but they are not easy to find. Before you buy any, you have to make sure the package is marked GF. Otherwise, the oats may be filled with gluten from contamination and must be avoided. Your best bet is to avoid all oats, unless they specifically state that they are gluten free.

Food Questions

Q. What can my child drink?

A. Milk alternatives can be good, if he or she has no intolerances for any of the ingredients. Water is always a great choice. I would avoid anything with caffeine for a child. Juices can be fine, but some children have problems with apple, berry, and other juices because of yeast or salicylate issues. If you serve juice, only serve 100 percent juice. Trial and error will tell you whether your child can tolerate the juices.

If your child does fine with fruit, try making smoothies. Put in a milk alternative, fruit juice, sorbet, and frozen fruit in a blender, and whirl it up. This is a good way to add calcium or protein powder, if needed. Whole Foods Market makes GFCF, non-artificial sodas under the 365 brand. Sodas are not a great beverage because of their sugar content, but once in a while, they can be fine.

Q. Is chocolate "milk-alternative" ok?

A. Yes, as long as extra sugar or chocolate are not problems. The companies add sugar to make the chocolate taste sweet.

Q. Is goat milk GFCF?

A. No. All mammal milk contains casein. Some children may not react poorly to goat milk, but most do, just like they do with cow's milk. You can always experiment. Write down when you give your child the goat's milk, and watch for a reaction or a change, especially once you stop giving it.

Q. If a recipe calls for buttermilk, how can we adjust this for the GFCF Diet?

A. Add lemon juice or gluten-free vinegar to your milk alternative of choice, and let the mixture sit for a short time. Then add it to your recipe.

Q. Is there a "cheese" that we can eat?

A. If you are avoiding soy, cheese alternatives are difficult to find. Almond and rice "cheeses" are on the market, but most contain casein, which makes them not okay to eat. Read the label to make sure any cheese alternative is casein free. Galaxy Nutritional Foods (http://www. galaxyfoods.com) makes a GFCFSF rice cheese in sliced form that comes in three flavors. It has baby-blue wrapping with the word "vegan" printed on a purple ribbon. (Beware: Galaxy also makes a rice cheese with casein in it. That label does *not* say vegan on it.) Follow Your Heart and Soymage soy cheese are vegan, meaning no casein. But your child must be able to tolerate soy to eat them.

Q. Is couscous OK on this diet?

A. No. Couscous is made from wheat.

Q. Do you have a great mock "macaroni and cheese" recipe?

A. Yes. This is a wonderful and fairly easy recipe. I adapted it from a recipe that another mom gave me. She adapted it from a cookbook.

For the milk alternative, you can use rice, soy, hemp, or almond "milk." You also can use coconut "milk," if it is gluten free, or DariFree potato milk. If possible, buy it in 8-ounce containers, as not to waste.

For the cheese, Soymage and Follow Your Heart are good brands. Make sure the product is labeled as vegan, because many soy cheeses contain casein. Vegan rice cheese from Galaxy Nutritional Foods is GFCFSF. For GFCF margarine, try Willow Run, unsalted Fleischmann's, Earth Balance, or the GFCFSF type available at kosher stores—or ghee.

GFCF Macaroni and Cheese

- 6 to 8 ounces milk alternative
- vegan soy or rice "cheese," frozen
- rice, quinoa, or corn pasta, any shape, as much as needed
- 2 eggs
- 3 to 4 tablespoons of GFCF margarine

Boil the pasta according to the directions. In another pan, melt the margarine and then stir in the alternative "milk," stirring constantly. Break up the frozen "cheese" slices and stir constantly. Add the eggs, and continue to stir until it looks creamy. Drain the pasta, add to the sauce, and enjoy.

Freeze or refrigerate any leftovers. When you reheat them, add more "milk" and margarine to make the mac and cheese creamy again.

Q. Rice Dream is listed as gluten free on the package. I heard that this is incorrect. Is it?

A. As of the time of this writing, if you call the company, they will tell you that their product contains barley, but just "a little." There is controversy regarding products such as Rice Dream, that meet the federal GF standard of containing no more than 20 parts per million (ppm) of barley, thus gluten. In August 2008, the FDA changed this regulation. For more on this regulation, see: http://www.gluten.net/FDADraftRuling.htm or http://www.cfsan.fda.gov/~dms/glutqa.html.

Q. I heard vanilla extract could have gluten in it. Is this true?

A. Distilled alcohol is used to make some vanilla extract. Experts state that the alcohol is burned off during the distillation process and the extract can be considered GF. When in doubt, always call the company. Do *not* use fake vanilla, called vanillin. It is derived from artificial ingredients. Whole Foods Market, Trader Joe's, and health-food stores have alcohol-free vanilla that is GFCF and natural.

Q. Some flavorings and extracts state on the label that they have alcohol in them. Is this okay?

A. Some grocery-store brands of flavorings use synthetic alcohol in their products. While this is GFCF, it is made from chemicals, something we always went to avoid. Health-food stores carry alcohol-free and often organic extracts. These types are wiser choices.

Q. Is wheat alcohol okay?

A. Actually, it is gluten free, because the distillation process removes the gluten.

Q. I heard that beer and some other alcoholic drinks are not gluten free. True?

A. You certainly will not be giving your child any alcoholic beverages. I have included this for adults who may be considering the diet for themselves. Most beers contain gluten, although there are GF beers on the market. The fermentation process does not remove the gluten. Some other alcoholic beverages made from gluten grains are also not allowed.

Q. What can we use for pancake syrup?

A. 100 percent maple syrup is best. There are two different forms, Grade A and Grade B. Some people prefer one over the other, so you will want to experiment. Some feel that Grade A syrup is much stronger and bolder in flavor than Grade B. Some people prefer to use agave nectar for syrup. You can make your own syrup by mixing brown and white sugar with water and then boiling until the mixture thickens. Add alcohol-free vanilla for flavor, if you want. I would stay away from grocery store brands because they are not maple syrup, but chemical-filled sugar.

Q. What lunch meats and hot dogs are safe to eat?

A. If you are watching soy, check the ingredients. Stay away from nitrites because they are not healthy. Here are some popular brands that are GFCF and nitrite and nitrate free: most of Boar's Head's meats,

Applegate Farms, Wellshire Farms, Shelton's, and Hormel Foods' Natural Choice line.

Q. How do I make GFCF, 100 percent natural hot dogs taste better and juicier?

A. Boil them for three to four minutes and enjoy. Some people think the beef ones are juicer than the turkey or chicken ones. Try Shelton's, Wellshire Farms, or Applegate Farms.

Q. My child cannot tolerate some other GF grains, such as potatoes and rice. What do you suggest?

A. Check out Nu-World Foods (http://www.nuworldfoods.com). Their products contain a grain called amaranth, which is GFCFSF. You can ask your store to stock the items you would like to try. If the store is not interested, you can purchase the items online. Amaranth has a large amount of dietary fiber, protein, iron, and calcium, as well as other vitamins and minerals.

As another option, consider corn products. Many items have corn as the grain. Flours from corn or beans can also be substituted for rice- and potato-based flours. Quinoa is another popular grain that is used in some pastas.

Q. Is Crisco shortening GFCF?

A. There is some controversy about butter-flavored Crisco, but regular Crisco is GFCF. However, it is not as healthy as Spectrum organic palm oil shortening, which comes in a tub at Whole Foods Market, health-food stores, and online.

Q. My son does not like the texture of many fruits. Is there another way to get him to eat fruit?

A. Yes! Smoothies. Use a blender or smoothie maker. Put in liquid ("milk" alternative or juice, or both), add frozen fruits and possibly sorbet. Whirl it up for a great treat. Add protein powder, calcium, or any other supplement you want your child to have. The mixture can be frozen in shapes as frozen treats, too. Also consider 100 percent fruit leathers (no sugar added) as a fruit alternative.

Q. Is cocoa butter GFCF?

A. Yes, just make sure there is *no* comma between "cocoa" and "butter" on the label. Cocoa butter is just the cocoa or chocolate part of the bean. If you see the comma, the product is *not* GFCF, because it contains butter from milk.

Q. Are baking powder and baking soda always gluten free?

A. You cannot always be certain. Many that are gluten free are now being marked as such on the label. If you are in doubt, call the company.

Q. Does lactic acid, sodium lactate, potassium lactate, or calcium lactate contain casein?

A. The Food Allergy & Anaphylaxis Network says that lactic acid, sodium lactate, potassium lactate, and calcium lactate do not contain milk protein and need not be restricted by someone avoiding milk. These agents are used as preservatives, mainly against yeasts and fungi. They are also used to increase the stability of antioxidants and to prevent the drying of different products.

Sodium lactate is produced by the natural fermentation of the sugars from corn or beets. However, lactic-acid starter culture may contain milk. Some experts state that it is produced commercially by the fermentation of whey, cornstarch, potatoes, and molasses. Yes, whey is dairy. Call the company when in doubt. Potassium lactate is a natural acid produced by bacteria in fermented foods.

Q. What about cream of tartar or calcium stearoyl lactylate? Do they have dairy in them?

A. No, they do not contain casein, or dairy.

Q. Besides being GFCF, my son also must be egg free. Help! What can he eat?

A. People who are vegan do not eat any foods connected with animals. This means no meat, no poultry, no seafood, no dairy, and no eggs. If you are looking for products or recipes without eggs or dairy, look for those marked "vegan." You can often use egg replacer (Ener-G brand) to substitute for eggs in a recipe. Vegans do eat grains, so make sure the product or recipe has no gluten in it. In recipes, change the flour to suit your needs to make it gluten free.

Religious Questions

Q. Communion wafers have wheat in them. Does a GFCF one exist?

A. Yes, Ener-G makes communion wafers that are vegan, GF, and soy free. Depending on your religion, you might want to discuss this option with your clergyperson. Some religions have different views on what is permissible.

Q. Can we find a GFCF matzo?

A. If you search online, you will find many recipes for matzo and matzo-related foods. Try all of the various spellings to expand your search: matzo, matzah, and matzoh. Gluten Free Matzos (http://www.glutenfreeoatmatzos.com) offers GFCF matzos made from gluten-free oats. The only ingredients are GF oat flour and water. The matzos can be ordered online from the British company and shipped to many countries.

Q. Is wheat starch gluten free?

A. Wheat starch is produced by removing proteins, including gluten, from wheat flour. Many years ago, wheat starch was thought to be safe for those on a gluten-free diet. However, it has been proven that removing all traces of protein is impossible and a small amount remains. Two types of wheat starch exist. The first, commercial wheat starch, is not suitable for those on gluten restricted diets. The second form is a specially manufactured type that is very expensive. It is permitted on the gluten-free diet in some European countries, but not in the United States. That is because the washing process is rarely complete, leaving residual gluten in the wheat starch.

Chapter 10

☞ **Menu Ideas** ☜

The most common question about the GFCF Diet is "What can my child eat?" This chapter is intended to serve as a handy reference guide at mealtime. Every food listed here refers to the version that is GFCF, dye free, and preservative free. Some of these items are available ready made, and some you will have to make from scratch or from mixes.

Many GFCF recipes are available in books and on websites. Also check: Yahoo Groups' GFCF recipe and support group (http://health.groups. yahoo.com/group/GFCFrecipes) or Delphi Forums' celiac disease online support group (http://forums.delphiforums.com/celiac/messages). Keep in mind that GFCF items may contain soy or other intolerances that your child must avoid.

Breakfast

- Pancakes
- Waffles, regular and Belgian
- French toast
- Eggs, hard boiled, soft boiled, scrambled, omelet-style, fried, over easy, or poached
- Egg salad
- Omelets mixed with meats, "cheeses," vegetables
- Frittatas with the same as above
- Soufflés

- Crepes
- Quiche
- Blintzes
- Strata
- Toast
- Bagels
- Muffins
- English muffins
- Biscuits
- Cinnamon toast or rolls
- Doughnuts
- Grilled cheese sandwich
- Cereal bars
- Sausages
- Bacon
- Ham
- Canadian bacon
- Breakfast burritos
- Potatoes
- Potato pancakes
- Cereal, hot and cold
- Fruit
- Smoothies
- Shakes
- Yogurt

Lunch

- Sandwiches, nut butter with or without 100 percent fruit jelly or jam, meat, poultry, egg salad
- Sandwiches made with waffles or rice cakes instead of bread
- Tortillas with "cheese," meat, other spreads
- Tortilla roll-ups or wraps
- Meat loaf
- Hot dogs
- Hamburgers or turkey burgers
- Chicken patties
- Chicken pieces
- Chicken salad
- Grilled "cheese"
- Beans
- Lentils
- Soup
- Quesadilla
- Tacos
- Burritos
- Taquitos
- Pizza
- Chili
- Rice bowl
- Meat salad
- Pasta and sauce, with or without meat or turkey
- Macaroni and "cheese"
- Meatballs and sauce, with or without pasta
- Chicken nuggets
- Leftovers from the night before
- Yogurt
- Nuts or seeds
- Chips

- Crackers
- Pretzels
- Rice cakes
- Fruit, fresh, dried, canned, or 100 percent leathers
- Trail mix
- Veggies, raw or cooked

- Snack bars
- Cookies
- Cake
- Brownies
- Muffins
- Pudding

Appetizers

- Crackers
- Paté
- Dips
- Spreads
- Seafood

- Chicken
- Beef
- Mini-sandwiches
- Meatballs
- Deviled eggs

Dinner

- Chicken
- Beef
- Lamb
- Fish
- Ribs, beef or pork
- Pork chops
- Pork loin
- Shellfish
- Spaghetti and meatballs
- Spaghetti and meat sauce
- Spaghetti and white sauce
- Pasta and ground turkey or beef
- Hamburgers
- Hot dogs
- Casseroles
- Meat loaf

- Tacos
- Pizza
- Rice bowls
- Soup
- Stew
- Chili
- Beans
- Pot pies
- Lasagna
- Manicotti
- Cannelloni
- Risotto
- Enchiladas
- Burritos
- Fajitas
- Salads
- Rice

- Potatoes
- Cornbread
- Bread or rolls
- Yams
- Squash
- Corn
- Vegetables
- Fruit
- Desserts

GFCF Meal Plan and Recipes

Here are menus for a two-week period, so you do not have to decide what to make each day. Recipes are included for items that are italicized on the menus.

Week One

Monday

- Breakfast: Waffles topped with fresh berries, orange juice, DariFree
- Lunch: Turkey sandwich, pretzels, wedges of pineapples, *Carrot Muffins*
- Dinner: Tacos with ground turkey meat, refried beans, rice, sorbet, DariFree

Carrot Muffins

- 4 4-ounce jars of organic carrot baby food
- 3/4 cup canola oil
- 2 cups white sugar
- 3 eggs
- 3 cups GF all-purpose baking flour
- 1 teaspoon cinnamon
- 1 teaspoon ground cloves
- 1/4 teaspoon ginger
- 1 teaspoon nutmeg

- 1 teaspoon GF baking powder
- 1 teaspoon baking soda
- 3/4 teaspoon salt
- 2 tablespoons ground flaxseed meal (optional)

Preheat oven to 400°F (205°C). Line baking cups, or grease with Spectrum vegetable shortening. Mix carrots, oil, sugar, and eggs in a large bowl. In a medium-sized bowl, mix flour, spices, baking soda, and baking powder. Add dry ingredients to carrot mixture and mix. Add flaxseed meal for extra fiber and omega-3 fatty acids (optional). Spoon into muffin cups. Bake 25 minutes or until toothpick comes out clean.

Makes 24 muffins. Eat some now, and freeze the rest for breakfasts or snacks.

—*Courtesy of Tori Tuncan (http://gfcfblog.blogspot.com); recipe adapted from Sarah Cook's pumpkin muffins at Autism Share (http://www.autismshare.com).*

Tuesday
- Breakfast: Cereal, DariFree, orange pieces
- Lunch: Taquitos, corn chips, apple
- Dinner: Spaghetti and meatballs in sauce, salad, *Blueberry Crepes*, DariFree

Blueberry Crepes

- 1 cup your favorite GF all-purpose flour mix
- 1 1/2 cups milk alternative
- 4 large eggs
- 1/4 cup melted margarine
- 3 tablespoons sugar

- 1/8 teaspoon salt
- blueberries
- MimicCreme, sweetened (It is GFCFSF.)

Mix the first six ingredients well. Pour mixture into a pitcher or other container with a pouring lip. Cover and let stand in the refrigerator for 30 minutes to 1/2 day.

Place a nonstick or seasoned crepe pan over medium-hot heat. Coat the pan with a little margarine. Stir the batter and pour a few teaspoons into the pan, lifting it off the heat and tilting and rotating it so that the batter forms an even, very thin layer.

Cook until the top is set and the underside is golden.

Turn the crepe over, using a spatula or your fingers, and cook until the second side is lightly browned.

Remove the crepe to a piece of wax paper. Continue cooking the rest of the crepes, greasing the pan as needed and stirring the batter before starting each one.

Stack the finished crepes between sheets of wax paper. To serve, fill each crepe with blueberries and top with MimicCreme. Use crepes immediately or let cool, put into large tightly sealed plastic bags and freeze. Leftover batter can be kept in the refrigerator for several days and then used.

—*Courtesy of Mireille Côté, at Delphi Forums' celiac disease online support group (http://forums.delphiforums.com/celiac/start) and restaurant owner, Granby, Quebec, Canada (http://casagranby.com/english/casa.html).*

Wednesday
- Breakfast: Pancakes, 100 percent maple syrup, melon, DariFree
- Lunch: Soup, crackers, fresh cherries
- Dinner: *Roasted Chicken*, potatoes, vegetable, fruit salad, DariFree

Roasted Chicken

- 6 cloves garlic, minced
- Whole fryer chicken
- 1 tablespoon dried basil
- 1 tablespoon dried marjoram
- 2 teaspoons salt
- 2 tablespoons oil

Preheat oven to 350°F (175°C). Mix all ingredients except chicken in a small bowl.

Put chicken, minus neck and giblets, in a roasting pan.

Starting at neck cavity, loosen skin from breast, drumsticks and thighs of chicken by inserting fingers and gently pushing between skin and meat.

Rub seasoning mix under loosened skin with fingers. (This is a bit messy but worth it, The meat, not the skin, is seasoned, and the skin keeps the meat from drying out in the oven.)

Bake for approximately 1 1/2 hours. Remove skin and serve.

—Courtesy of Alison from Autism Share (http://www.autismshare.com).

Thursday
- Breakfast: Scrambled eggs, breakfast sausage, toast, DariFree
- Lunch: Soy yogurt with fresh fruit, snack bar
- Dinner: *Chicken Pot Pie, Carrot Muffin,* fruit cup, DariFree

Chicken Pot Pie

- 1 pound boneless, skinless chicken breast halves, cubed
- 1 cup sliced carrots
- 1 cup frozen green peas
- 1/2 cup sliced celery
- 1/3 cup margarine
- 1/3 cup chopped onion
- 1 can mushrooms, drained*
- 1/4 cup cornstarch
- 1/2 teaspoon salt
- 1/4 teaspoon black pepper
- 1/4 teaspoon celery seed
- 1/4 cup dry parsley
- 1 3/4 cups GF chicken broth
- 3/4 teaspoon GF concentrate or dry chicken bouillon
- 1/3 cup dry sherry or other liquid
- 2/3 cup milk alternative
- Crust (see recipes below)

*Freeze the mushroom water to use later when you make stock.

Preheat oven to 425°F (220°C).

In a saucepan, combine chicken, carrots, peas, and celery. Add water to cover, and boil for 15 minutes. Remove from heat, drain, and set aside.

In the saucepan over medium heat, cook onions in butter until soft and translucent. Add all liquids except for 1/3 cup reserved in a small jar with a lid. Add cornstarch to the 1/3 cup liquid, and shake the closed jar. Add to the rest of liquid and veggies. Mix and add, pepper, parsley, and celery seed. Remove from heat and set aside.

Place the chicken mixture in the bottom of the dish. Pour the hot liquid mixture over it. Cover with the crust (see recipes below). Make several small slits in the top to allow steam to escape.

Bake in the preheated oven for 30 to 35 minutes, or until pastry is golden brown and filling is bubbly.

Cool for 10 minutes before serving.

For single crust:
- 1 cup basic GF mix
- 2 tablespoons sweet rice flour
- 1/4 teaspoon salt
- 6 tablespoons cold unsalted margarine
- 1 egg
- 1 tablespoon cider vinegar or lemon juice

For double crust:
- 1 1/2 cups basic GF mix
- 3 tablespoons sweet rice flour
- 1/4 teaspoon salt
- 9 tablespoons cold unsalted margarine
- 1 jumbo egg
- 1 1/2 tablespoons cider vinegar or lemon juice

Basic GF flour mix (makes 3 cups)
- 1 cup chickpea or garfava flour
- 1 cup brown rice flour
- 2/3 cup potato starch
- 1/3 cup tapioca flour

Mix together the GF mix, sweet rice flour, and salt. Cut margarine into chunks and, using fingertips or a dough cutter, work the margarine into the dry ingredients to form a coarse meal. Make a well. Break the egg into the well. Add vinegar or lemon juice. Use a fork to stir from the center, working the flour into the egg to form a soft dough. Shape into a flat cake. Cover and refrigerate if too soft to roll out.

To prebake a pie shell, preheat the oven to 400°F (205°C). Use the single-crust recipe, and roll into a round 10" to 12" in diameter (depending on the size of the pan). Grease the pie plate, spring form, tart pan, or quiche dish, and fit crust into pan. Flute the edges, and bake 12 to 15 minutes or until golden brown. Generally, pie weights are not needed for GF pastry.

—Courtesy of Mireille Côté.

Friday
- Breakfast: Hot rice cereal, toast, juice with calcium
- Lunch: Hot dogs cut up with barbecue sauce, potato chips, raw carrots, fruit
- Dinner: Chili, cornbread (365 brand), sugar-snap peas, cookies, DariFree

Saturday
- Breakfast: Omelet, juice with calcium
- Lunch: Burgers, raw vegetables, fruit, cookies
- Dinner: Chicken skewers, green beans, brown rice, *Impossible Chocolate Pie*, DariFree

Impossible Chocolate Pie

- 2 eggs
- 1 cup milk alternative
- 1/4 cup margarine
- 1 teaspoon vanilla
- 2 ounces melted chocolate
- 1 cup GF brown sugar
- 1/2 cup GF "Bisquick" mix

Preheat oven to 350°F (175°C). Put everything into a blender and blend for 1 minute. Pour into greased pie plate. Bake for 30 minutes or until tests done with knife. Cool completely.

GF "Bisquick" Mix (to keep on hand)
Works well for all "Bisquick" recipes, except biscuits.
- 2 1/2 cups rice flour (could be white, brown, or half and half)
- 1 2/3 cups potato starch
- 3 teaspoons baking powder
- 2 1/2 teaspoons salt
- 2 tablespoons sugar
- 1/2 cup DariFree powder (http://www.vancesfoods.com)
- 3 tablespoons egg replacer powder
- 1 cup less 1 tablespoon shortening

In a large bowl, whisk together all dry ingredients. Cut in the shortening until no lumps appear. Store mix in the refrigerator or freezer, due to shortening in mix.
　　Note: for the above recipe, use only 1/2 cup of this mix.

—Courtesy of Mireille Côté.

Sunday
- Breakfast: French toast topped with fruit, juice with calcium
- Lunch: Chicken nuggets, raw vegetables, applesauce
- Dinner: Homemade pizza (Kinnikinnick crust, tomato or spaghetti sauce, rice cheese, toppings), salad or cut-up vegetables, melon, DariFree

Week Two
Monday
- Breakfast: Poached eggs, toast, juice with calcium
- Lunch: Grilled "cheese" sandwich, corn chips, fruit leathers, peaches
- Dinner: Grilled turkey burgers, corn on the cob, tater tots, *Fruit Crisp*, DariFree

Fruit Crisp

Topping Mixture:
- 6 tablespoons GF "Bisquick" mix (see recipe above)
- 1/4 cup light brown sugar, packed
- 1/4 cup granulated sugar
- 1/4 teaspoon ground cinnamon
- 1/4 teaspoon ground nutmeg
- 1/4 teaspoon salt
- 1/4 cup (1/2 stick) margarine
- 3/4 cups pecans, walnuts, or whole almonds, chopped coarse (or chopped fine if mixing topping by hand)

Fruit Mixture:
- 2 1/2 to 3 pounds fruit of choice (See below for ideas.) (~6 cups cut up)
- 3 to 4 tablespoons granulated sugar (more as desired)
- 1 1/2 tablespoons fresh lemon juice and 1/2 teaspoon grated lemon zest from one lemon

For Apple Crisp:
Cut up equal quantities of Granny Smith and McIntosh apples. Peel, core, and cut apples into one-inch chunks. Cut up 6 apples for about 6 cups.

For Apple-Raspberry Crisp:
Follow recipe for Apple Crisp above, reducing the amount of cut apples to 5 cups (about 3 medium Granny Smith and 2 medium McIntosh) and adding 1 cup rinsed fresh raspberries to fruit mixture.

For Peach-Blueberry Crisp:
Follow recipe for Apple Crisp, reducing amount of cut peaches to 5 cups (about 5 medium peaches) and adding 1 cup rinsed fresh blueberries and 1 tablespoon quick-cooking tapioca to fruit mixture.

Half a teaspoon of grated fresh ginger makes a nice flavor addition to all of the fruits.

For the topping: Place GF "Bisquick" mix, brown sugar, sugar, cinnamon, nutmeg, and salt in a food processor fitted with a steel blade. Add nuts, and pulse until mixture resembles crumbly sand, about five 1-second bursts. Do not overprocess, or mixture will take on a smooth, cookie-dough texture. (To mix by hand, allow margarine pieces to sit at room temperature for 5 minutes. Add margarine; toss to coat. Pinch margarine chunks and dry mixture between fingertips until mixture looks like crumbly wet sand. Do not overmix.) Refrigerate mixture while preparing fruit, at least 15 minutes.

Toss cut-up fruit, sugar, lemon juice, and zest (along with 1 tablespoon quick-cooking tapioca if using blueberries) in medium bowl.

Adjust oven rack to lower-middle position, and heat oven to 375°F (175°C). Scrape fruit mixture with rubber spatula into 8-inch square (2 quart) baking pan or 9-inch round deep-dish pie plate. Distribute chilled topping evenly over fruit; bake for 40 minutes. Increase oven temperature to 400°F (205°C); bake until fruit is bubbling and topping is deep golden brown, about 5 minutes longer. Serve warm or at room temperature.

To make a larger crisp that serves 10, double all the ingredients, use a 13 x 9-inch baking pan, and bake for 55 minutes at 375°F (175°C) without increasing the oven temperature.

—*Courtesy of Mireille Côté.*

Tuesday

- Breakfast: Cold cereal, DariFree
- Lunch: Hot dogs, beans, chips, fruit
- Dinner: *Chicken Wraps*, brown rice, fruit salad, DariFree

Chicken Wraps

- 1/4 teaspoon salt
- 1 1/2 cups Bob's Red Mill all-purpose GF baking flour or other GFCF flour
- 1 tablespoon shortening
- 1 large egg
- 1 to 1 1/2 cups of water
- 1/2 to 3/4 cup shredded chicken (per wrap)
- Mild or hot sauce, as desired
- Vegetables, as desired

Mix flour, salt, and shortening until crumbly. Then mix in egg, and add enough water to make batter very soupy. Pour 1/2 cup of batter into a lightly greased pan on medium-high heat. Cook for 30 seconds to 1 minute on each side. Add chicken and other ingredients, as desired, into each wrap. Roll and eat.

Makes 5-6 servings.

Freezes well. To thaw, just microwave for 30 seconds.

—Courtesy of Sarah from Autism Share (http://www.autismshare.com).

Wednesday

- Breakfast: Bagel with peanut butter, DariFree
- Lunch: Taquitos, snack bar, tortilla chips, fruit leather
- Dinner: Sautéed (pan-fried) chicken with garlic, baked potatoes, string beans, *Baked Pineapple*, DariFree

Baked Pineapple

- 2 tablespoons cornstarch
- 1/4 cup water
- 2 eggs, beaten
- 1 can (15 1/4 ounce) crushed pineapple, undrained
- 1/2 cup sugar
- 1 teaspoon vanilla
- margarine
- ground cinnamon

Combine cornstarch and water, and stir until smooth. Add eggs and blend well. Add pineapple, sugar, and vanilla; mix well. Pour into a lightly greased 1 1/2-quart casserole dish, dot with margarine, and sprinkle with cinnamon. Bake at 350°F (175°C) for 1 hour.

—Courtesy of Mireille Côté.

Thursday
- Breakfast: Hard-boiled egg, toast, juice with calcium
- Lunch: Turkey sandwich, Tings corn snack, snack bar, fruit
- Dinner: Fish sticks, *Scalloped Potatoes*, salad, DariFree

Scalloped Potatoes

- 6 medium boiling or baking potatoes (~2 pounds)
- 3 tablespoons margarine
- 1 small onion, finely chopped (1/4 to 1/2 cup)
- 3 tablespoons GF all-purpose flour mix (or potato starch)
- 1 teaspoon salt

- 1/4 teaspoon pepper
- 2 1/2 cups milk alternative

Heat oven to 350°F (175°C).

Spray a 2-quart casserole dish with non-stick spray.

Peel potatoes and cut into 1/8-inch slices to measure about 4 cups.

Melt 3 tablespoons margarine in saucepan over medium heat. Cook onion in margarine about 2 minutes, stirring occasionally, until tender. Stir in flour, salt, and pepper. Cook, stirring constantly, until smooth and bubbly; remove from heat. Stir in milk alternative. Heat to boiling, stirring constantly. Boil and stir 1 minute.

Spread potatoes in casserole. Pour sauce over potatoes. Cover and bake 1 hour. Uncover and bake 30 to 45 minutes longer, or until potatoes are tender and top begins to brown. Let stand 5 to 10 minutes before serving. Serves 4-6. Best served hot out of the oven, but fine left over.

Notes: Choose the size of casserole dish based on the number of people you want to feed and use the amount of potatoes necessary to fill that dish. Increase all the ingredients proportionately. I usually use about 8 to 10 potatoes, 1/2 cup of onion, up to 1 1/4 teaspoon salt, and around 3 cups of milk alternative.

—*Courtesy of Jennifer Riordan, Delphi Forums' celiac disease online support group (http://forums.delphiforums.com/celiac/messages/?msg=49402.1)*

Friday

- Breakfast: Cereal, DariFree
- Lunch: Chicken sandwiches, pretzels, applesauce
- Dinner: *Pineapple Shrimp in Sweet and Sour Sauce*, white rice, DariFree

Pineapple Shrimp in Sweet and Sour Sauce

- 1 pound shrimp, shells removed
- 2 tablespoons GFCF soy sauce
- pepper, as desired
- 4 carrots, thinly sliced
- 2 ribs of celery, sliced
- 1 onion, in cubes
- 1 green pepper, cut in 1/2" to 3/4" cubes
- 1 red pepper, cut in 1/2" to 3/4" cubes
- 1 fresh pineapple, cubed

Sweet & Sour Sauce:
- 3 tablespoons sugar
- 1 cup tomato sauce
- 1/4 cup GF vinegar
- 1 1/2 tablespoons cornstarch
- 1/2 cup juice of pineapple
- 1 tablespoon fish sauce

Put shrimp in a bowl with soy sauce and pepper, and mix. Sauté shrimp, and add vegetables. Add sweet and sour sauce mixed with cornstarch (make a slurry with the cornstarch before adding), and let simmer until thick and transparent.

—Courtesy of Mireille Côté.

Saturday
- Breakfast: *GF Apple Pancake Bake*, 100 percent maple syrup, DariFree
- Lunch: Fajitas with corn or brown rice tortillas, rice, beans, fruit
- Dinner: Barbecued turkey breasts and legs, sweet potatoes, corn, DariFree

GF Apple Pancake Bake

- 4 to 5 baking apples (depends on size of apples and pan; McIntosh are best)
- Cinnamon and sugar to taste
- Double recipe or batch of your favorite GF pancake mix (e.g., Bob's Red Mill)

Preheat oven to 350°F (175°C). Line a baking sheet (with ~1 inch sides) with foil. Spray with GFCF nonstick spray.

Peel apples, cut, and remove seeds. Cut apples in thin slices (like you would for an apple pie, but thinner because they cook for less time and you want them to get soft).

Toss apples with cinnamon and sugar (to taste). Line bottom of pan with single layer of apples.

Prepare pancake mix (double recipe) according to directions. Add a few sprinkles of cinnamon and sugar if you want. (You don't need to, and be careful it doesn't get too sweet.)

Pour pancake mix over the apples. (Mix comes to about the top of the side of the cookie sheet.) Sprinkle the top with cinnamon and sugar to make it look nice.

Bake for 15 to 18 minutes, or until brown on top and cooked through. (I've never had a problem of it not cooking all the way through.)

Serve warm with or without 100 percent maple syrup. Also good later in the day as a snack— you can zap it in the microwave oven to warm it, but it's still good at room temperature. This is not very good the next day, I'll be honest—the pancake part gets a bit too dry for my tastes.

—Courtesy of Jennifer Riordan.

Sunday
- Breakfast: Omelet, hash browns, toast, DariFree
- Lunch: Chicken salad with balsamic vinegar, chips, fruit

- Dinner: *Crockpot Chicken Cacciatore*, garlic bread, squash, fruit, DariFree

Crockpot Chicken Cacciatore

- 2 cups fresh mushrooms, sliced
- 1 cup celery, sliced
- 1 cup carrot, chopped
- 2 medium onions, sliced or cut in wedges (but not too big)
- 1 green, yellow, or red sweet pepper, cut into strips (use as many as you want)
- 4 cloves of garlic, minced (or 4 to 5 teaspoons of prediced garlic packed in water)
- 1 to 2 pounds of boneless chicken breasts, cut in large pieces (if breasts, thighs, or drumsticks, skin and use 3 pounds)
- 1/2 cup GF chicken broth
- 1/4 cup dry white wine (or chicken broth, which is what I use)
- 2 tablespoons quick-cooking tapioca (or a thickener like corn-starch mixed with water)
- 2 bay leaves
- 1 teaspoon dried oregano
- 1 teaspoon sugar
- 1/4 teaspoon salt
- 1/4 teaspoon pepper
- 1 14.5-ounce can of diced tomatoes (not drained)
- 1/3 cup tomato paste
- GF pasta, cooked and drained

Combine mushrooms, celery, carrot, onion, peppers, garlic, and chicken in the crockpot. (If you have chicken pieces with bone, place those on top of the veggies.) In a bowl, combine the broth (or wine and broth), tapioca, and spices. Pour over chicken, and cook on low for 7 hours or on high for 3.5 to 4 hours.

If on low heat setting, turn to high after 7 hours. Add the undrained tomatoes and the tomato paste. Cook on high for another 30 minutes. Salt and pepper to taste.

Serve over hot, cooked GF pasta.

Notes: If you don't have quick-cooking tapioca, add a mix of water and cornstarch along with the tomatoes. This will thicken it. Do this anyway if you think it needs to be thicker. If you like more tomatoes, add 2 cans.

I never use white wine. Just substitute the same amount of stock, and it's good.

I like to use boneless, skinless pieces when I'm serving this to guests—it is a lot neater and easier to eat.

—Courtesy of Jennifer Riordan.

Chapter 11

Dealing with Naysayers

Through the years, I have run into many people who have negative things to say about the GFCF Diet. The most common comment is that someone tried the diet and it just did not work.

Yet, so often when I've spoken with people who have told me that they thought the diet didn't work, I discovered that they had not followed it correctly. They did not understand that it has to be followed 100 percent of the time and that it has to include toiletries, art supplies, cosmetics, and more. They also did not comprehend the importance of keeping food and other items safe from cross-contamination.

In addition, they did not recognize that the diet takes more than simply removing gluten and casein. Other foods might also need to be removed, especially those containing dyes and preservatives—and perhaps phenols and salicylates as well. In some cases, children cannot experience the positive effects of being GFCF because they have yeast issues or intolerances for soy or other foods.

Sometimes the only way to see the full impact of the GFCF Diet is to eliminate the other foods that disagree with your child. Also, you may need to add supplements or enzymes, or combine this diet with another, listed in Chapter 13, to see the complete benefits of the diet.

So many doctors coax parents into giving their children drugs to combat problems instead of looking at what the child is putting into his or her body and how that could cause the inappropriate or challenging behaviors and symptoms.

Parents need to be proactive for their child's sake. Questions have to be asked. If parents do not get the response that they think is right from their child's doctor or medical practitioner, it is time to move on. The science of medicine is not easy, but it should not take a "one size fits all" approach.

Not all doctors think alike. Getting a second or third opinion has proven successful for many people. Remember that you are in charge of your child's body and your own. You have the right to explore other options and other thoughts and ideas. Be open to listening to opinions from a variety of medical experts and then make the best decision for you and your family.

You will find that food companies rely on artificial additives, which generally are extremely profitable and far cheaper than using real food to color their products. Many of these food companies also use television commercials or print ads to coax children to buy this or that cereal or fruity candy. Healthy products are not advertised.

Parents believe these advertisements, too. Do not fall into this trap. Know that these foods are unhealthy for your children and their bodies, as well as your own bodies. Parents need to watch for reactions in their children's behaviors and not blame the children. Many inappropriate behaviors are the fault of what children are being fed by their parents! Often, it is not the child's fault for behaving unruly, loud, out of control, nasty, or vicious. The food they are given is making their minds and bodies react in what most parents would see as an unacceptable manner.

Many parents tell me that their child does not react to certain foods, when they most certainly do. The problem is that many parents are not paying attention to the signs. Document, observe, keep a journal, and be aware of how your child is really behaving. Here are some signs and behaviors to consider.

- Is he or she having nightmares?
- Night terrors?
- Does he or she have trouble sitting still?
- Does he or she have a lot of eczema?
- Other skin disorders?
- Asthma?
- Bowel problems?
- Meltdowns?
- Violent behaviors?
- Stimming?
- Is he or she biting or hurting other children?
- Does he or she chew on his or her clothing?

These behaviors may actually be food related. Stop being a naysayer. Pay attention to what you are feeding your child. Real the labels, write the ingredients down, and watch for reactions.

If you could avoid medications by eliminating foods, wouldn't you want to give it a try? What if changing what your child eats makes him or her be able to sit still, behave appropriately, be pleasant to be around, and become more of a typical child? Is this not what everyone wants?

Never be afraid to ask questions. The Yahoo Groups' GFCF Kids message board (http://health.groups.yahoo.com/group/GFCFKids/messages) is full of messages from parents who believe in the GFCF Diet and other interventions that have helped their children. These parents all started out like you—confused, bewildered, and overwhelmed. They can help answer any questions that perhaps this book did not address. Remember, the only silly question is an unasked one. Bookmark this site, and you'll have a source of help.

Chapter 12

Success Stories from All over the World

When I first was investigating the gluten-free, casein-free diet, I came across a story in *Parents* magazine by Karyn Seroussi titled, "We Cured Our Son's Autism," written in 2000. It opened my eyes, gave me hope, and empowered me to try the diet for my son. You can read the story at the magazine's website (http://www.parents.com/parents/story.jsp?storyid=/templatedata/parents/story/data/2085.xml).

Since I've begun working with the GFCF Diet and advocating for it, people the world over have contacted me for help with the diet and to share their success stories.

I do not like the terms "cured" or "recovered," because I believe that autism is a lifetime disorder. However, many parents, including myself, still believe that this diet can help greatly in improving, erasing, and reversing many autistic traits and symptoms—often with other interventions also incorporated. Following this diet can and does help remove many autistic traits.

If they were evaluated after being on the GFCF Diet, many children would not be diagnosed with the level of autism that had been part of their previous lives. They might just receive a diagnosis of pervasive development disorder not otherwise specified (PDD-NOS). This means they may have traits of autism so slight that only a trained professional or a knowledgeable parent would notice.

Is this diet still a success without effecting a cure? Absolutely! Imagine an onlooker who hears that your child is autistic. Yet standing before him, he sees a typically developing child who behaves like all of the other children surrounding him or her. The onlooker comments about being shocked by your "autistic child." That is all you need to hear to know that you, too, have a success story. When you have a success story, tell the world. Scream it from the rooftops. Email everyone on earth. Spread your glory!

Parents find success stories essential to help them keep going, give them hope, provide promises for the future, and allow them to persevere in fulfilling their dreams of having a healthy, happy child who is very close in behavior to other typically developing children.

This chapter brings you the stories of eight mothers of children with autism spectrum disorders, as well as one child and one woman with Asperger syndrome. I hope their successes will give you the hope you need to pursue the diet and achieve your dreams of a better future for you, your child, and your family.

Julie Czechowski, Virginia

It seems like forever since I started the diet. Six years ago, I would read the Yahoo GFCF Kids message board several times a day. It was a lifeline to someone starting out on the GFCF and autism journey. Eventually, as I discovered the recipes that I needed and became adept at making my own GFCF meals for my son, I visited the board less and less.

My son had been diagnosed with Asperger syndrome. I started him on the diet when he was six-and-a-half years old. That is old, considering that a lot of people these days are starting far earlier. When we started the diet, we unfortunately did not see immediate, dramatic results. That was discouraging, but we kept at it, and I was very strict about infractions. Slowly, very slowly, we began to get results. But it wasn't until we added the Feingold Stage II Diet, removing foods high in salicylates, such as apples and tomatoes, that we finally got our dramatic results. His gut improved significantly, he gained weight, and things started to roll for us.

Of course, we also did a slew of other treatments (under the supervision of a doctor associated with Defeat Autism Now!) including chelation, treatment for yeast, and vitamin supplements. Five years later, our doctor told us that my son's stomach had healed enough for us to try gluten and dairy infractions to test his behavioral and neurological reactions. Unfortunately, our experiment was a disaster, and it was painfully obvious that his body was not quite ready for it.

But, one year later, we tried again, and this time we met with success.

This does not mean he is off either the GFCF or the Feingold diet. We plan to stay with both for the foreseeable future, and any changeover will be extremely slow. But it did mean he had a regular piece of pizza with his classmates to celebrate a peer's birthday and didn't freak out or look stoned. During the summer, he ate a couple of regular pieces of birthday cake with ice cream.

And every now and then, he's allowed to actually eat the bun with his McDonald's hamburger. We tried these non-GFCF foods very carefully. Our doctor suggested the following schedule. For six weeks, include one gluten infraction per week. Just one. That means one piece of bread, one cookie, or one something with gluten for the entire week. So you'd have six carefully planned and observed infractions in six weeks.

Then take a one-week break from gluten infractions and start a four-week infraction period with dairy. Same thing, except no straight glasses of milk or milkshakes because that would be too much. Apparently only four weeks is needed for the dairy because symptoms will present themselves quicker and more obviously physically, in the form of runny stools or runny noses, rather than neurologically.

The first time we tried a gluten infraction (and mind you, this was after five years of super-strict GFCF and Feingold Stage II), it was a disaster. My son became hyper like crazy and even developed a voice tic. And this was just after one gluten infraction for the whole week! Sigh. We never even got to the dairy part. One year later, it's a different story. Why? I'm not sure; I guess his tummy just wasn't completely healed yet. And "completely" is the key word here. Even so, it's staggering to think that his stomach needed six, long, freaking years to heal completely. And even then, we aren't sure it's completely, completely healed, if you know what I mean!

What I'm trying to say is that, once their stomachs have improved, some kid can expand their diets to include gluten and dairy without suffering neurological reactions. My son is so used to the GFCF Diet now that other stuff actually tastes funny to him. So I sincerely believe that, as he gets older, he'll largely stay GFCF by choice. But I wanted to write this to give all you newbies hope that healing does happen if you stick with the diet, even if you don't see immediate, dramatic results.

Melinda Alleyne, Olathe, Kansas

It's Never Too Late for an Older Child

Our son's story is typical of so many.

Joshua developed normally until his vaccinations at eighteen months old, when he rapidly spiraled out of control. Within three days, our son was lost to us. Our once sweet and loving boy was replaced by a child who no longer wanted us to touch him—who now screeched, banged his head, giggled for hours, and wouldn't sleep longer than two hours, ever. Sadly, Joshua no longer liked his favorite toys, preferring to sit and rock, or to run wildly around in circles. His sweet disposition was replaced with violent seizures.

For months we muddled through life looking for answers on our own. We tried everything we knew to try and recover our son, praying that as he got well, he would get better—but little help was available in 1994. At best I got sympathetic looks from doctors that mostly said: "Give it up, lady. No help is out there for your child. You just have to learn how to accept it. He was *born* autistic"…"You just never saw the signs"…"It's just coincidence"…and so on.

I never gave up hope.

Thankfully the Autism Research Institute existed and I had the privilege of talking with and being encouraged by Bernard Rimland, PhD, in those early days before he started Defeat Autism Now! At Dr. Rimland's suggestion, we tried a gluten-free, casein-free diet. We tried melatonin, vitamin B6 and magnesium, dimethylglycine, trimethylglycine, and music therapy—the list could go on and on. We tried ABA, PECS, TEACCH and good ol' "discipline" to no avail.

We took Joshua to countless "specialists" across the nation, and yet his seizures were relentless and his behavior was hideous. We spent thousands of dollars. He was evaluated at Keesler Air Force Base (home of the second-largest medical facility in the U.S. Air Force), at Emory Center for Autism, at the Judevine Center for Autism, and at Philadelphia Children's Hospital for studies in Landau-Kleffner syndrome.

We even tried taking our son to see Defeat Autism Now! physicians during their formative years. Anyone remember IV secretin for seven hundred dollars a whack? Yes we did that, too—twice a month for an entire year. Joshua painstakingly improved through the years, but we were constantly reminded that most of his improvements were minor, and our financial debt was great. He was grossly behind in all skills and was increasingly self-abusive, intolerably aggressive, and without any functional language. He was still severely affected by autism.

When he was fourteen, we took Joshua to yet another doctor, just hoping he could help Joshua to stop cutting himself. He was so severely lost in self-abuse that it wasn't uncommon for him to have gaping, pus-filled sores all over his skin. We decided to revisit the Defeat Autism Now! concept of biomedical healing. We had tried this in its early years, eventually becoming discouraged with it because it didn't seem to be helping. But we were now desperate.

Joshua was tested this time for food allergies and intolerances. The results showed many, many intolerances and several environmental and food allergies. Once we removed these foods from his diet and he became free of gluten, casein, soy, and corn, miracles literally started to happen in his life. Our son spoke for the first time by the fifth day on his new diet... and was off all psychiatric medications within the first two months. As time went on, we added several nutritional supplements, started chelation, and began giving him MB12 shots. Thankfully, his body was finally ready to receive these treatments that had failed before. He was finally healing from a lifetime illness brought on by his vaccines.

This time, we got the miracle we had been praying for. Day by day, Joshua is returning to us. He now has functional language (around three hundred or more words). During this past year, he has learned to make his bed, clean his room, do household chores, ride his bike, skip, jump rope, do puzzles, and play games. Two weeks ago, he played with the neighborhood children for the first time ever, while I watched and cried.

He is learning to enjoy pastimes that, just a year ago, would have gotten us hit, had we even suggested he try them. Daily, he is becoming more a part of our family. He is learning to write, and his academic skills have soared these past few months. Joshua also is making his own choices about what he wants to do and how he wants his room to look, for the first time ever.

Just as stunning are the things that Joshua is no longer doing. He no longer makes spit pictures over all the windows in our house. The walls of his room are no longer painted with his poop during the night. He no longer just lies around wanting to do nothing all day except rip up every book in the house. He no longer fixates on certain movies or on us all having to wear shoes.

All of his sleep and eating issues are now resolved. He no longer is self-abusive or aggressive. He is off all psychiatric medicines and is being weaned from his seizure meds. He no longer self-stims constantly, and the hysterical giggling is gone. He is no longer severely affected by autism.

Every day is simply a new miracle. Our son is now mildly to moderately affected by autism. And more healing comes with each and every day. I am glad we never quit believing that healing could and would someday happen. In my humble opinion, it is never too late.

Melinda Alleyne runs an online military support group called: Living with Autism and in the Military (http://health.groups.yahoo.com/group/autismandmilitarylife).

Rachelle, New Zealand

At this point, I think we're definitely having some success with my eldest son, George, who is language delayed but not ASD. His speech has blossomed on the diet; he's almost five years old and starting primary school in the new year. My youngest, Ian, who is three years old, is babbling more and has started to say small words, like "up," "please," and "go." He also is more interactive. My husband is not convinced that this is because of the diet, though he is willing to admit that being on Efalex (fish and evening primrose oil combo) has improved our son's eye contact, reduced his stims, and improved his mood by a large amount!

George was born weighing 9 pounds, 9 ounces, and had low blood sugar due to my lack of breast milk. He was put on supplemental feeding until my milk came in six days later.

As he grew older, we noticed that he was not talking like his contemporaries. We asked our doctor to refer him for hearing and other tests. George was talking, just not in English. You could hear sentences in the cadence. He did speech therapy privately, which made a small difference, but he was getting frustrated and started hitting some of the other kids.

Ian was born via ventouse (vacuum extractor) after his heart rate dropped and then rallied just before they were going to do an emergency c-section. He was a strong baby, but not overly happy. He grew normally, but he was very quiet and grizzly. I asked the doctor to refer him earlier than I had done with George because Ian was showing no signs of speech. When he eventually started talking, he said one word—once and then never again.

Both boys had the meningococcal C vaccine after the medical professionals pressured me into it. The vaccine didn't affect George, as far as we could tell, but Ian stopped trying to talk completely. He went silent, stopped looking at us, and started ignoring us. He began following lines, running with his head to the side, and showing a number of other abnormal behaviors.

About this time, we finally got to the assessment process, and in May 2007, Ian was diagnosed as being autistic. During the initial assessment, he had no eye contact, was not interested in any of the activities in which they wanted him to participate, and spent the time climbing onto the tables and jumping off onto me.

We had started Ian on Efalex shortly before the diagnosis. It took a couple of months to see results, but gradually he changed into a happy child. We got much more eye contact, and his autistic behaviors mostly disappeared. He started babbling a bit and was a bit easier to deal with in Kindy (school in New Zealand for children ages three to five or six).

At the beginning of September 2007, we started going gluten free. Within two months, George's speech improved a great deal. Kindy has commented on it, as have a number of other people. He still has days where it's not so great, but this is becoming less common. Ian has increased his babbling and is starting to include small words in his vocabulary. Both boys are less frustrated at Kindy, and Ian is now interacting with the other kids sometimes. He has even joined other children on a few occasions as they play spontaneously and is improving all the time. I am not maintaining a casein-free diet at the moment, but we may try it again later. It's hard enough getting my husband to work with our boys being gluten free. Being casein free is much harder.

Casein-free foods are rather hard to find unfortunately here in New Zealand. We can only get rice, soy, and almond milk. DariFree and hemp milk aren't here. I've only found one CF butter substitute; it's expensive and doesn't taste that great. Ghee is available, but that's also expensive. There are plenty of oil choices, though. I use rice bran oil for baking if I'm cooking or baking dairy free. (My sister-in-law is allergic to dairy, so I have to make cakes that she can eat, too.) Oil didn't work in biscuits, though; it tasted wrong.

Gluten-free foods are expensive but easier to find. I get most of my flours from my local Asian supermarket. I buy rice, tapioca, potato, buckwheat, chickpea, jowar (sorghum), maize, and corn flour on a regular basis. I use these for making our own bread because I'm not prepared to spend six dollars or more per loaf, and the boys don't think much of the bought stuff anyway.

I do some baking and will be doing more, because the ready-made biscuits are expensive. We use store-bought pasta that I get from either the supermarket or the Asian supermarket. I'm doing a lot of label reading because I want to reduce soy as well. I can still use some of the foods we used to have, like tinned (canned) tomatoes, baked beans, and other tinned vegetables. Being gluten free is a lot more expensive, but that's partly because I'm still finding new things that we can try. Last week, for example, I found sweet potato pasta. I think we're starting to reach the point that I know what's working for us. I'll continue getting that stuff and not get the other things that didn't work. I'm considering getting a food dehydrator to make my own fruit wraps. I already have a pasta maker that I've cleaned thoroughly, as well as a bread maker. I got a new toaster, too.

The downside is that Ian is going through a fussy phase of only liking potatoes, chips, corn (sometimes), and pasta. That makes things rather hard, but he doesn't seem to be suffering from it.

Recently both of my boys have shown reactions to gluten that Kindy noticed when I forgot to warn the school about the boys' possible reactions to gluten foods. My husband continued to be against the diet until recently, because he had not seen any proof. He has become supportive since Kindy has noticed changes in my boys when they have had reactions to foods with gluten. Ian only had a small gluten infraction at a barbecue at my brother's place, but he went back to running around in a circle at Kindy. George had a double infraction and got a bit aggressive, which is not normal for him at Kindy.

I think there is great value in talking with your husband and letting him know how much you need his support. If he undermines your efforts when he is out with the kids, that makes you feel frustrated and sad. I found that it helped a lot with our issues when he realized how bad it was making me feel.

Hopefully that gives you an idea of how things are going.

Natalie, Nova Scotia, Canada

In spring 2003, our son Connor, age four, was diagnosed with moderate autism.

Connor was nonverbal, had little or no eye contact, did not acknowledge peers at day care, did not respond when spoken to, and did not feel pain. He also had chronic diarrhea, was an extremely picky eater, slept only two to five hours each night, took no naps, and was hypersensitive to high-pitched noises like those of a vacuum or hairdryer. However, he loved to hug. He would climb into any adult's lap for a hug and was very independent about getting what he wanted or needed.

I was devastated by the diagnosis, of course, and went through a period of denial. I was thinking, "Autistic kids don't like to be touched!" But Connor loved to be cuddled.

I decided that I needed to spend more time with him. I was able to get a leave of absence from my job after my doctor wrote a note recommending that I receive a leave for stress. I was able to get off work for two-and-a-half months. The only thing that we achieved during that time was getting my son potty trained.

That fall I also attended my first autism seminar. At my second seminar, in March 2004, I purchased a book called *Freaks, Geeks, & Asperger Syndrome* by Luke Jackson. Luke was thirteen when he wrote this book. He mentioned the gluten-free, casein-free diet in the book and how much it had helped him and his family. This interested me. I went to the Autism Resource Centre near me and took out every book I could find on the subject.

I found *Unraveling the Mystery of Autism and Pervasive Development Disorder* by Karyn Seroussi to be fascinating. I read the entire book in two days. I learned so many things.

At the end of April 2004, I put Connor on the GFCF Diet. We went cold turkey. (This is not recommended—especially with older kids because they can experience severe withdrawal symptoms for several weeks.) Of course I didn't know that at the time, but fortunately Connor had such a dramatic improvement within the first week that I was encouraged enough to continue and figure out exactly what worked best for him.

Several people will agree with me, including Connor's speech therapist, Kim Trefrey, childcare providers, my family, and many friends.

Connor suddenly began to take an interest in his speech therapy sessions, began to interact with peers at day care, felt pain, and responded when spoken to. (Mind you, the response was usually "Nooooo!" at that point.) He also began to have normal bowel movements.

After two to three weeks on the diet, however, he started displaying hyperaggressive behavior. He had never done this before. I went back to my research and was referred to the Feingold Diet by other parents on the GFCF Kids forum on the Internet. I began to eliminate artificial substances, such as colors, flavors, sweeteners, and MSG. We also had to eliminate certain fruits for Connor, such as concentrated apple products (sauce or juice), red grapes, and bananas. We could only allow limited amounts of berries, citrus, and cocoa, as well as limited amounts of preservatives, especially nitrates and sulfites.

The frustrating and difficult part of diet intervention is that children react differently to foods as varied as the autism spectrum itself. You have to figure out what works best for your child. My best advice is to keep a daily diary. Use one page per day. You will begin to see trends. Only add or remove one type of food or supplement at a time and wait a week before adding another new one. This will prevent confusion and save you time in the long run.

I know that the diet sounds very difficult and confusing. In the beginning it is, but now after three years, it is second nature. I basically cook like my grandmother used to—from scratch. I use unprocessed meats; fresh, frozen, or canned vegetables; fresh or frozen fruit; some canned fruits; and pure herbs. I do not spend astronomical amounts on groceries. In one month, I spent ninety-one dollars on specialty foods. Considering that I don't buy ready-made foods with artificial ingredients or preservatives and that we don't eat out often, the cost works out to about the same as other families' budgets.

Now, after three years on the diet, Connor can speak in full sentences, has good eye contact, sleeps through the night (most of the time), initiates play with peers, responds when spoken to, and is no longer sensitive to high-pitched noises. He even vacuums! He eats a wide variety of foods and is within the average height and weight for his age.

The diet is not a cure for autism. I believe it is responsible for the first 50 percent of Connor's progress, because it opened his mind to being able to learn. The other 50 percent, I attribute to the wonderful team at his school.

It is our job as parents to participate actively in the IPP sessions and educate ourselves. We know our children better than anyone else and what does and doesn't work for them. Read, attend seminars and meetings, listen to everyone, and sort out what makes sense for your child.

If something gives you a sick feeling in your gut, say no, even if the idea was recommended by a professional. If you feel something is worth a try and might work for your child, insist on it. Many teaching techniques are based on sound theories, but the facilitators can make a difference. If they really care, they will find the right combination for each child. We have the right and the responsibility as parents to make those decisions.

Joyce Chicoine, Albany, New York

My son, Joe, was nonverbal and had several symptoms of autism fifteen years ago when he was three years old. We are fortunate that we live where we do, because he was able to start receiving special education, speech and motor therapies without having a formal diagnosis.

Joe also had several health problems, including asthma and chronic fluid in his ears. Prescription medications only seemed to make him worse. We took him to a highly recommended allergist, who did regular allergy testing and concluded that Joe was allergic to pollen, dust, and animal dander. This allergist said Joe wasn't allergic to any foods or molds. Yet, when we started Joe on the allergy treatment that this doctor recommended, his symptoms continued to get worse and he needed even more medication.

I decided it was time for a second opinion. So I took him to an ear-nose-and-throat specialist and allergist who did a radioallergosorbent blood test (RAST) to check for allergies. The RAST showed that *Joe* was allergic to several types of mold and eighteen of the twenty foods that were tested.

I thought, "Who do I believe? Is this blood test accurate?" I did a little research and learned that the RAST is not highly accurate if the results are negative. But if the results are positive, it's fairly reliable. Since Joe's results were mostly positive, we knew that we needed to do something. Eliminating the eighteen foods that he reacted to was out of the question—a diet consisting of codfish and baker's yeast (the only two foods he didn't react to) would not be very nutritious, to say the least.

The second doctor told us that he couldn't treat Joe's numerous food allergies (long story), so we ended up taking him to another doctor out-of-state. This doctor did a different type of allergy testing called intra-dermal provocation-neutralization testing. The testing is expensive and time-consuming but makes it possible to set precise treatment doses for each allergy that can be administered under the tongue at home (instead of going to the office for allergy shots). By the way, the intradermal P-N testing confirmed the results of the RAST.

The third doctor also told us that it's not normal to have so many food allergies and sensitivities. (You think?) He suspected that Joe had a "leaky gut" and that something was damaging his intestine—probably either gluten or a buildup of a yeast called Candida. The doctor did some blood tests and concluded from the results that gluten *was* indeed the problem.

That was more than fourteen years ago, long before the GFCF Diet was a popular alternative treatment for autism. The only book I knew then about the diet was written by a mom of autistic triplets living in western Massachusetts. She figured out on her own that her autistic children were suffering from a metabolic disorder that prevented them from digesting gluten and casein properly.

Joe has been on the GFCF Diet for more than fourteen years. (We decided to eliminate milk because it was one of his worst allergies.) He finally got his formal diagnosis of Asperger syndrome when he was in kindergarten. The developmental pediatrician who made the diagnosis chose to ignore my son's significant speech delays or he would have diagnosed him with autism instead.

I don't think that the GFCF Diet is a cure-all, but it certainly has helped my son to respond more positively to other sorts of sensory and educational treatments. The sensory treatments that Joe had included sensory integration with an occupational therapist, Berard auditory integration training with an audiologist certified as a Berard practitioner, and vision therapy with an optometrist who was a Fellow of the College of Optometrists in vision development. Joe was in regular classes throughout his thirteen years of public schooling and gradually had almost all of his special services eliminated because he no longer needed them. Throughout middle and high school, the only service he received was social work and the only modification he had was double time allowed for tests.

Joe is now a freshman in college and has been getting along well living in the dorm with a roommate. He takes honors classes and even made the Dean's list his first semester. He is majoring in political science and hopes to go to law school after he graduates from college. Joe chooses to stay gluten free and casein free because he believes that he feels better and functions better when he stays on the diet.

Petra van Meeteren, the Netherlands
Alex's Story

Mom
Alex was twelve years old when he finally received an official diagnosis of Asperger syndrome. The long road that led to this diagnosis had been difficult for him.

In school, other kids did not accept him, so the remedial teacher suggested social skills training. In first grade, Alex stopped reading after the first four months of starting to read. The remedial teacher said Alex was dyslexic. In the next grade, they gave him extra lessons for that, all repetition.

In third grade, they never mentioned dyslexia again because he was reading above his grade level. I think this had to do with the subjects of the books. The books in third grade actually had subjects in them that interested him. His grades were okay, but we knew that he was very smart. We told his teachers that, but they responded that he just didn't show them. So we had him tested.

Still nothing came out of that, though the psychiatrist later told us that Alex fit the autism profile perfectly. He had very high scores in logical parts but extremely low scores on the parts on communication. We could add many more issues like this that were easily explained by school, such as saying that he was just a slow kid. My gut instinct told me that there was more to it, and I finally took him to the pediatrician who diagnosed Asperger syndrome.

Now that we had a diagnosis, we started to gather information about autism. We started going to meetings with other parents who had teenagers with autism. Many of them had the same story. We then found out about a book called *Freaks, Geeks, & Asperger Syndrome* by Luke Jackson. Alex finished the book in two days and started asking about the diet. I had already looked into this and found numerous websites on the subject.

We decided to try it for six months. This was in January. We took milk from his diet because this was the easiest. I felt I needed to get more information about gluten. We went gluten free and casein free in February. Around the middle of March, we started noticing a dramatic change in Alex. We went from the twenty-minute, early-morning ritual of trying to get Alex out of bed to Alex waking up his dad! There was no need to remind him of all the things that he needed to do before heading out the door. Amazingly, he started to feel better, too! He had more energy and was more focused. We are hoping that his grades will pick up, too.

Alex also noticed that the annoying tic that he had (he kept saying the letter G) was gone. Actually, most of his tics are gone. When he received his report card, he was disappointed at the grades. Usually this would end up in a long night of crying and overall depression. This time he cried for five minutes and went on with his business. At dinnertime we have very nice conversations now, without having to remind Alex constantly to let his brother finish talking or that he should not have comments on every subject. We're not there yet, but I am sure that he will improve even more because I still find hidden ingredients in certain foods.

Besides removing gluten and milk from his diet, we started him on probiotics and vitamins. We visited a nutritionist to confirm that Alex is getting all the nutrition that he needs at his age. It is a shame we don't have doctors associated with Defeat Autism Now! here.

Alex's migraines have increased; this is something we are monitoring. They could be due to stress. He is not accepted in class, and that causes a lot of stress. Perhaps puberty has to do with it. But overall the diet has had a major impact on Alex's behavior, and we will continue to stay on it as long as Alex is motivated to do so.

Alex

Before I knew that I had Asperger syndrome, I felt different than other kids. The guys in my class did not accept me because of that. I didn't watch *Pokemon* because I just didn't see the point of it. I did not share their interests, and so they did not accept me. This was very difficult for me. Also in class, I didn't understand some of the stuff the teacher was talking about. But I could not make them understand why I didn't understand.

Last summer my mom took me to get tested for autism, and getting the diagnosis made me understand that other people may not always understand me because I think in a different way. Getting my point across is very hard, that is why I am having my mom help me write this story.

I started the diet after I read the book from Luke Jackson. I realized that the diet was really helping him and that I should try it, too. My mom took away milk, then gluten. At first I did not feel any different. But after four weeks, I noticed that I was better focused when I took a test in class. I also started feeling better, and this I noticed during my hockey practice.

We are now four months into the diet, and my mom also took MSG out of my diet. The bad part about this diet is missing out on Mars bars and cheese! But my mom is a good cook and she has even made pizza taste like pizza.

By writing this story, I hope I can help other kids. My mom is talking about making a website to help kids in the Netherlands. There is not much information about the GFCF Diet over here. This diet could really help kids on the autism spectrum, and I hope parents will support them like my parents do me.

Phyllis Zimmerman, Colorado

When parents first hear the word "autism," a part of their world dies. Dreams that were wrapped in the baby blanket of potential are shattered into a thousands shards of painful glass that cut to the core of the parent's heart. Sadness gives way to despair as they hear the supposed limitations of their child's intellectual capacity and ability to function in a normal world. Everything modern pediatrics had to say about autism in 1999 was discouraging.

Our grieving process began but was interrupted with hope and promises that we felt we received from God's word. We clung to the promises that there is a plan for Anthony's life, plans that will help him prosper and not to harm him, plans to give hope and a future. This promise gave me a new mindset. My dreams were not dead; my son was not dead. Neither my son nor my dreams needed to surrender to the disorder of autism. Through divine leading and healing, we would redefine the dreams and discover the fullness of who Anthony Zimmerman was becoming.

The journey to bring about hope and a future for our son started with the implementation of the gluten-free, casein-free diet. In 1999, the information was limited and prepared foods were almost nonexistent, so I began the task of making GFCF foods from scratch. Bette Hagman, the "gluten-free gourmet," became my teacher and mentor through her vast experience with gluten-free cooking and baking for those with celiac disease.

We started with the removal of casein first. That was easiest since we did not drink much milk or use milk products. The harder task was to remove the gluten and soy products. We were vegetarians, and soy was a staple. Because our son reacted to soy, we had to shift our lifestyle and add organic, free-range poultry and buffalo to his diet.

Following the removal of gluten and casein over a two-week period, we heard the word "Mommy" for the first time. Small improvements were made as we continued on the journey of hope and a future.

In addition to the diet, we took my son to the Pfeiffer Treatment Center (http://www.hriptc.org) and found that he suffered from leaky gut and malabsorption, rendering his body unable to absorb the vitamins and minerals he needed for proper mental development. We had been on the GFCF Diet for a few months, so we had already started the first line of treatment to restoring his gut issues. We then started vitamin, mineral, and supplemental treatments to improve the leaky gut and malabsorption issues. With the combination, greater gains were seen.

During the six months of dietary intervention, I read everything I could get my hands on and decided to attend my first Defeat Autism Now conference. I was amazed, shocked, and empowered by the findings physicians presented and started down an even more precise course of treatment. Every treatment protocol they discussed started with the GFCF Diet! I knew I was on the right course and continued with a deeper biomedical understanding of what we were doing for our son.

Sleeping through the night, potty training, and educational and social goals were reached on an almost daily basis. Anthony and I worked hard together on applied behavior analysis (ABA), relationship development intervention (RDI), and speech at home. The combination and hard work were paying off, and we were rewarded with a renewed hope and future. Our dreams shifted and were redefined as our son flourished under the biomedical and behavioral treatments.

The journey started six years ago in 2002, and we all have grown in leaps and bounds. I have had the opportunity to attend six Defeat Autism Now! conferences, start a support group called Dietary Interventions Support and Hope (DISH), and help hundreds of parents navigate the beginning of this often confusing journey. I have reaped so many rewards personally and have grown significantly in my own personal development. It has become my mission to assist and educate physicians, parents, teachers, and caregivers about the benefits of diet interventions for those on the autism spectrum.

As for my son Anthony, he is doing great! He was initially diagnosed as being moderately affected with autism, placing him in the middle of the autism disorder spectrum. Today he is considered high functioning and very close to recovery. We keep pressing forward to the hope and future God has promised us for him. We continue to share with others what the ancient Greek physician Hippocrates noted hundreds of years ago: "Let food be your medicine and medicine be your food."

If you would like more information about DISH, contact Phyllis Zimmerman at ascl@autismlarimer.org.

Saswati Singh, Dehra Dun, India

The Impossible Dream

As the saying goes, "The impossible dream can only be attained in possible stages." I have seen this manifested in the lives of so many of our very special children, with whom I had the extreme good fortune to interact and serve, even from my school days. As the secretary of the Social Service Club in School in Kolkata, I served daily with Mother Teresa and her Missionaries of Charity. Little was I to suspect that in my middle years, when I ultimately said "yes" to marriage, I would be blessed with the most special gift of my life!

My son, Prasanna (name changed) sits today in his favorite sofa, viewing his mates. They are friends who are like his brothers—and all call him Bhai, which means "brother." When I look at all of them, it seems that they have known each other from earlier lives. This innocence, clarity, and untold love are so eloquent! And evident.

In my long journey of twenty years with Prasanna, he has taught me so much. Patience—which I had very little of. Insight—a lot of which I have now been able to culture. Understanding—this is still growing with each breath! And so much more. He and all of this have enriched my life. Without him, I would have lived and died like the normal run of teachers.

I have been asked over and over by different people—friends, relatives, well-wishers, and journalists—to write about my experiences with the Inspiration Group Home. So, I sat down to write about how I ultimately came to start this group home with my son and other children from our school in Delhi who are now young adults. Some parents come to take their children home once a week or once a fortnight. Some go home every night. It all depends on the family situation and needs.

With the sound microbiological and genetic background at Presidency College, Kolkata, I had the natural inclination to look at the reasons behind everything. Likewise, when our children showed bizarre behavior or were not able to stay calm, I tended to delve into the possible reasons. Was it some intrinsic factor? Was it due to some extrinsic factor? Did something happen in the morning to which he was showing a delayed reaction? In most cases, I realized, my son's behavior had to do with some sensory stimulation.

This is where behavior therapy, occupational therapy, sensory integration, speech therapy, and alternative therapies all came to my rescue. Here too, the factor of previous preparation was a sure success. For example, all of the boys had problems with hair cutting and nail cutting, which was addressed with this technique.

I attended the Son-Rise Program Start-up in 2003 at the Option Institute in Sheffield, Massachusetts. When I returned home, I did not blindly start the program, but I started by changing my son's diet to the recommended GFCF one. I believed in the holistic approach, and as I started to phase out the milk and wheat, I noticed that the first reaction was the elimination of his extremely severe constipation. Prasanna was already 15 years of age, too far gone, I had thought, to start the diet!

This brings me to the very interesting topic of diet therapy. With the GFCF Diet, my son showed immediate improvement. Prasanna calmed down a lot and became more focused, and his eye contact improved. He was able to speak more relevantly, and the aggression was subsiding. This allowed us to stop all of his medication for hyperactivity and calmness. Presently he is only on anti-epileptic drugs.

As I tried all this with him, I also tried to see whether it would hold good for the others, as well. The first hurdle was to convince the parents of the children in the group home. A few agreed. As I have always taken one step at a time, we used the same technique. We gradually phased out the milk, as this takes about a month to flush it out from the system. Along with this, we stopped the sugar. Then gradually we cut out the wheat, one product at a time, over a month or two, depending on individual cases.

Along with this, we introduced ragi (as it is popularly known in South India) or marwah (as it is called in North India), which is black millet. Millet is high in calcium and protein, and supplies the products that are eliminated in the diet. The diet has to be followed religiously, and only then we can start seeing a gradual change. Sometimes, the change is quite dramatic. But the kitchen has to be monitored by a trained person.

Prasanna had developed severe jaundice four years back, which could have been be due to the long-term administration of anti-epileptic drugs. This left his digestion shattered and his health in ruins. But it taught me a lot about digestion and diet therapy. He is presently GFCFSFSF—that is, sugar and soy free, besides being gluten and casein free.

When he developed severe reflux esophagitis, the pediatrician advised us to get his allergy tests done. To my chagrin, Prasanna proved to be highly allergic to rice also! Even now we are struggling to balance his diet with the help of the top nutritionists in Delhi. When we tested him for urine porphyrin in France, we found three heavy metals—mercury, arsenic, and lead! With his poor health, we did not dare to do chelation, so as an alternative, we grind mint and coriander leaves (commonly used in India to make chutney) into his food, which has the chelation effect. We are also giving him chlorella.

Prasanna's case was an eye-opener. When we did the tests for the others, six of them had very strange results. Two boys were allergic to potato, another to apple and baker's yeast, and many to ticks and mites. Nearly all of them showed high dust allergy. To counter this, we started to use the vacuum cleaner to kick off less dust in the premises. Washing with water was another option.

Most of the children are able to sit at the computers for short stints. They have learned to sight-read their names, because they type their names in different colors every day. The diet therapy has improved their concentration. Most of the children who were underweight have gained weight, as much as 12 kilos (26 pounds), in one case. But the diet is followed only in the case of children who have allergies, and only when the parents are approving.

My repeated advice to parents is: do not give up hope. "Never Despair" is the Inspiration motto. This factor alone has helped me in going forward—step by step.

I know for a fact that "the impossible dream can only be attained in possible stages."

Emma Hasenstaub, Bellevue, Nebraska

I am thirty-five years old, and I have Asperger syndrome. I always knew that I was different from the others when I was a child. The other children would be off playing with each other, and I would be sitting in the corner with one of my books. Part of it was that I was very short for my age, and people generally thought that I was a lot younger. Once they heard me speak, they were often a little baffled. I remember hearing parents say that they were surprised that I was so articulate, and my teachers often commented on my vast vocabulary.

I always got along very well with adults, whether they were parents or teachers, but I never seemed to know what to talk about with the other kids. I felt like I was an adult trapped in a child's existence.

In early elementary school I suffered from horrible headaches and stomachaches that were dismissed as anxiety or nervousness. With the stress of moving to a new town and attending a high school full of strangers, I felt sick all of the time. There were some foods that I just couldn't stand the texture of, like rice and pasta and oatmeal, but because my sister was such a picky eater and considered such a pain, I kept my feelings about these foods to myself and ate them even though they disgusted me.

When someone did try to befriend me, I never knew what to say and generally said something that would end in me being teased and seen as very strange. I often stared off into space, and I never looked into people's eyes. One of my teachers asked me why I never made eye contact. I was convinced that it was because I grew up with a blind mother and it wasn't something that I was really taught to do. At the time, it seemed a plausible explanation.

One thing that I noticed was that when I stopped eating meat, some of my odd behaviors lessened a little.

Near the end of my first year of college, I was put on medication for my anxiety and depression, but I reacted very poorly to the medications and could no longer distinguish reality.

This went on until I was twenty-four years old, when I finally had a moment of clarity while switching from one antidepressant to another. I told the doctor that I was done taking the evil pills.

At this point, I noticed that every time I ate dairy products, I became more agitated than usual and that it was really making me feel sick. For a while, I attributed it to medication withdrawal, but after a year, I figured out that it really seemed to be dairy products. Once I eliminated dairy from my diet, I started to feel a bit more able to deal with everyday upsets. If I ingest dairy products accidentally, I cannot form coherent thoughts and sound like I am babbling.

After reading some articles on animal rights, I decided to eliminate eggs from my diet, and again, I found that some of my odd behaviors diminished. Eggs had more of a physical (gassy) effect than any mental or behavioral effects, though I think that it is important to acknowledge that the physical effects can really impact one psychologically.

I was proud of myself for graduating summa cum laude in my undergraduate studies and later being accepted to a PhD program in philosophy with a one-year fellowship, so I accepted. I was finally starting to feel like I could have a decent, "normal" life, but I had a very difficult time navigating the social networking part of the graduate program and had to drop out. Stress was a constant factor, and I was getting physically ill a lot again after I ate. What the heck could it be this time?

After keeping a food journal for about three months, I eliminated wheat from my diet. I began to lose weight and had to be hospitalized for a week to become medically stable. The staff was getting very upset with me because of my unwillingness to eat dairy, eggs, or wheat, so they decided to test me for food allergies and celiac disease.

I tested allergic to milk, chocolate, and eggs, but the test for celiac was negative. I explained to them that I felt better when I did not eat wheat, but I still felt a little off after eating certain foods and presented them with a list. My therapist said that it sounded like I was gluten intolerant and that I should avoid it.

At this time, I had read some literature on Asperger syndrome and asked my therapist about it. She said that it made a lot of sense since the diagnosis of social anxiety and depression never quite seemed right for me and because I was so awkward around other people. Additionally, she cited my awkward postures, self-stimulating behaviors, dislike of change in routine, and food sensitivities as additional support for the diagnosis. A psychologist set me up with an appointment for a formal evaluation.

Finally, I was formally diagnosed with Asperger syndrome.

If I was still eating gluten, I think that I would be a lot less able to cope with life than I am now because I would be physically ill along with being stressed out. It is a little challenging when people want to go out to eat because of the dietary restrictions, but I actually prefer to cook.

I do, however, keep a list of restaurants with "safe" items listed in case someone does want to go out spontaneously, and I appreciate that more and more chain restaurants are willing to provide ingredient listings for their foods. There is some legwork involved, but it is worth it to be part of what's going on rather than always hanging out on the fringes and *wishing* that I could be a part of the group.

The restricted diet can be frustrating, so I try to have fun with it. I enjoy changing "regular" foods into gluten-free vegan ones. The alternative is not an option for me. I am thankful to not feel the way I used to any more. We all have issues with certain foods. Some of us just have more severe cases.

My social skills have improved, too. I am able to go to church sometimes and talk with one or two people after the service. I can even go out and have coffee with people and converse. My life is the most "normal" that it has ever been, and people who have known me for years have commented on my improvement.

I hope that these stories provided you with hope, encouragement, and belief. Each story is so different, just like our children on the autism spectrum. Every child is different; every family is different; and every process or intervention is different. There are thousands of other success stories out there. Intervention does work! You have to search out what works best for your child. Do not give up! My hope and dream is that everyone who reads this book will be able to write his or her own success story one day. Keep reading. More help is on the way.

Chapter 13

≫ Other Interventions, ≪ Services, and Diets to Investigate

One size does not fit all. I am not talking about clothing. I am talking about the GFCF Diet and other interventions. Many children can benefit by going beyond the diet and receiving other behavioral and therapeutic interventions. Many children also benefit by having yeast overgrowth treated and nutritional deficiencies compensated.

Some children have positive results when enzymes or supplements are added into their diet. Some children benefit when phenols and salicylates are removed, as well as other allergens or intolerances. Some parents feel chelation is necessary if testing shows that the child has a high level of heavy-metal toxins. Some children can also benefit from other types of dietary protocols, as outlined in this chapter.

Bottom line: do nothing until you consult with a licensed medical practitioner or appropriate therapist or behaviorist. You might want to refer to the Defeat Autism Now! information in the Introduction to this book.

The services listed in this chapter, and other beneficial services that might be accessible where you live, might be effective. You may also be eligible, through various agencies, to obtain paid respite care, diapers, medical assistance, counseling, assistive technology devices, referrals to other agencies or resources, IEP advocacy or advice, letter writing, or perhaps financial assistance with day care.

Your child does not have to be of school age to receive services in the United States. Services can begin at birth for children with disabilities. Early intervention is the key, and the U.S. Individuals with Disabilities Education Act can help you.

Allergy Testing

Some families prefer to have blood and urine tests performed before beginning the GFCF Diet or other interventions. If you do this, your child should still be ingesting gluten and casein when the testing is performed. Keep in mind that allergy testing will check simply for allergies and generally not for intolerances. (Yet there are tests for intolerances, so consult with your doctor.)

Many children are indeed allergic to certain foods and other sources. If this is the case, take note of the other foods that your child should avoid, as well as gluten and casein. If you have testing performed and everything comes up negative, your child can still benefit from following the GFCF Diet.

Many parents choose to use Great Plains Laboratory (http://www. greatplainslaboratory.com) or Genova Diagnostics (http://www.gdx. net), formerly Great Smokies Diagnostic Laboratory, for the testing of their children. These labs test not only for allergies, but also for a host of other factors that can affect your child. Testing can involve gastrointestinal assessments, immunology assessments, nutritional assessments, endocrinology assessments, and metabolic assessments.

Ask your insurance company if it will cover the charges. Great Plains' and Genova's websites have information on which insurance companies cover their services. Some do, and some do not. If your insurance company will not cover these laboratory fees, consider printing out a list of the tests that these laboratories perform and sharing it with your medical practitioner. He or she may be willing to request the same tests from an insurance-covered laboratory. Note that many of these specialized tests are not performed at the average laboratory. Doctors who've attended Defeat Autism Now! conferences often use Great Plains and Genova because they specialize in testing for children with ASD, ADHD, and other disorders.

Therapies

Autism therapies can encompass an assortment of interventions, many of which can be very costly. Some services can be provided free through your school district. You can learn about them by contacting the district's special education department or school personnel at your local school district.

You should also be able to acquire a list of outside agencies to contact for assistance in obtaining help for your child. If your child qualifies for an agency's services, the agency can make him or her a client and share more details about services for free or at a low cost with government assistance.

Some interventions that have brought ASD children success include: occupational therapy, vision therapy, art therapy, speech and language therapy, sensory-motor integration therapy, therapeutic horseback riding and hippotherapy, listening therapy, neurofeedback, social skills training, functional behavioral analysis, applied behavioral analysis (ABA), discrete trial teaching (DTT), pivotal response training (PRT), and relationship development intervention (RDI). Some of these therapies include behavioral intervention, toilet training, and assistance with play dates and daily living skills. More websites on interventions are listed in the Resources section at the end of this book.

Here is a more detailed rundown on some of the various therapies.

Occupational Therapy

The American Occupational Therapy Association (http://www.aota.org) offers the services of occupational therapists (OTs) who assist children with special needs with daily tasks and life skills such as: getting dressed, motor skills (both gross and fine), visual skills, oral motor skills, other learning skills, sensory processing skills, handwriting skills, and playing with other children.

An OT will first evaluate the child for difficulties or delays with specific age-appropriate tasks. Then the therapist will help the child to improve skills that he or she lacks, or needs assistance with, through better use of the hands, wrist, legs, and arms. This can include help with dexterity, coordination, and strength.

Handwriting is often very difficult for children with ASD. It is a complex process in managing written language. This difficult-to-maneuver task requires coordinating the eyes, arms, hands, pencil grip, letter formation, and body posture. An OT can also help with other tasks, such as adjustment to various types of clothing textures or food textures, or facilitating with other sensory overload difficulties.

Sensory-Motor Integration Therapy

An occupational therapist usually facilitates this therapy. Sensory-motor integration therapy involves activities such as swinging in a hammock, balancing on beams, and brushing or stroking the child's body. The therapy works on the child's nervous system. The OT can help coordinate the movement of the child's eyes, head, and body. This therapy can help the child to maintain muscle tone, coordinate both sides of the body, and hold his or her head upright. As part of the therapy, the OT also can help the child become comfortable in dealing with all of his or her senses.

Vision Therapy

Vision therapy improves a child's visual efficiency, thus helping to correct visual-motor or perceptual-cognitive deficiencies, or both. Optometrists who choose this specialized field have had great success in treating individuals with learning-related visual problems, lazy eyes, computer vision syndrome, double vision, or convergence insufficiency. Visual therapy also can provide nonsurgical treatment of strabismus (eye turns or crossed eyes) and help with visually related reading difficulties and the visual parts of ADD behaviors.

Vision therapy does *not* focus on strengthening the eye muscles. Visual-motor skills and endurance are improved through the use of computer equipment and optical devices—such as therapeutic lenses, prisms, and filters. Visual therapy can help children to focus better, to have their eyes work together better (teaming), to read more effectively, and perhaps be able to stop wearing glasses. The therapy also can help with visual processing and improve overall vision. Having vision difficulties recognized and improved can improve the child's behavior and emotional well-being.

Optometrists who are board certified in vision therapy have successfully helped children with special needs, including developmental delays, visual perceptual visual-motor deficits, ADD, and ASD. To see if your child may have vision problems that could be helped by vision therapy, go to Optometrists Network (http://www.children-special-needs.org/parenting/eyesight_eye_care.html) and take the quiz.

For more information about vision therapy, visit the websites of the Optometric Extension Program Foundation (http://www.oepf.org/Patients&ParentsHome.php), the College of Optometrists in Vision Development (http://www.covd.org), or Parents Active for Visual Education (http://www.pavevision.org/).

Art Therapy

Art therapy combines psychological therapy and art to assist clients with: anxiety, depression, and other mental and emotional problems, as well as with addictions, family and relationship issues, and social and emotional difficulties related to a disability, disorder or illness, trauma, or loss. This approach also can help with physical, cognitive, and neurological problems, and psychosocial difficulties related to medical illness.

This creative form of therapy uses art to improve and develop physical, mental, and emotional well-being. The art therapist can help the person to find meaning through his or her drawings, paintings, collages, and clay designs. The art therapist emphasizes learning skills, developing and expressing images that come from inside the person.

An art therapy session focuses on the experiences, feelings, and ideas of the individual and concentrates on his or her perceptions and imagination. Through artwork, the client can express specific feelings that perhaps cannot be spoken or revealed in other ways. The art therapist can then do an assessment and create a treatment plan to help the client regain improved mental health.

Speech and Language Therapy

In speech and language therapy, a speech and language pathologist assesses the patient's needs in one or more areas of communication, including: articulation (sound and word production, so that speech can be understood), stuttering, voice (pitch, volume, and quality), receptive language (comprehension), and expressive language. Expressive language encompasses vocabulary, sentence structure and meaning, grammar and pragmatics, and the use of language in various social settings. Speech and language therapy can help with swallowing skills and provide treatment when necessary.

Therapeutic Horseback Riding and Hippotherapy

This form of therapy, also called equestrian or equine therapy, can be best explained as horseback-riding therapy for those with mental and physical disabilities. Riders learn horsemanship skills, including controlling and caring for the horses, if they are physically capable. These skills can increase the child's self-esteem, as well as improving his or her physical difficulties. Riders also learn to use their muscles, which helps them to maintain their balance. Riding horses helps build muscle strength, balance, postural control, and coordination. It also assists with increasing joint mobility and perceptual skills.

Listening Therapy

Alfred Tomatis, MD, an ear, nose, and throat specialist in France, pioneered the concept of listening therapy. Guy Berard, MD; Stephen Porges, PhD; Bill Clark; and Ingo Steinbach, PhD, have followed, each with their own concept of what a listening therapy program should entail.

Listening therapy is sometimes called auditory training, auditory stimulation, auditory integration training (AIT) or audio-psycho-phonology (APP). Besides the Tomatis approach, other listening programs include EnListen, the Berard method of AIT, and the BGC method of AIT.

This therapy involves listening to specific, guided music. The program is designed to re-educate the way a person listens to improve learning and language abilities, communication skills, creativity, and social behavior.

Listening therapy has been successful in helping people who need to have instructions repeated, are easily distracted or restless, daydream, have poor attention and concentration in learning situations, and misinterpret what is being said. Any of these problems can produce odd reactions and make communication difficult.

Listening programs have helped thousands of children with autism, auditory processing problems, dyslexia, learning disabilities, ADD-ADHD, and sensory integration and motor-skills difficulties. These programs also have helped adults fight depression, develop better communication skills, and improve creativity and on-the-job performance.

Listening training starts with a test that measures frequency responses, the ability to discriminate sounds, and ear-dominance. A detailed interview with the parents completes the assessment. Following the interview, a program is designed and a number of sessions set up to meet the individual's specific needs.

Each session consists of ear stimulation via the electronic listening device. This consists of a set of high-frequency-range headphones with an impedance of 150 ohms and a frequency range of 22,000 or 23,000 hertz, a microphone, and a system of electronic gates that filter sounds to specific frequencies. Parents and teachers usually report great changes in communication and behavior shortly after the first session. They also notice an increased motivation to learn and improvement in reading, writing, and concentration. Further listening tests confirm the changes.

Some listening therapy programs can be performed at home, with the use of a computer, headphones, and a CD.

Neurofeedback

Neurofeedback, also known as EEG (electroencephalogram) biofeedback or neurotherapy, is brain exercise or training in self-regulation. For neurofeedback, a professional in the field records brain waves after attaching special sensors to the client's scalp with EEG paste. The procedure is painless and noninvasive because it does not use any voltage or current to the brain. The sensors are attached to the scalp with the hair intact, so there is no need to shave the child's head.

After the sensors are affixed, a computer processes the brain waves and extracts information from the sensors. The ebb and flow of the brain waves and the specific information obtained is then shown to the client in the form of a video game. The client receives instructions on how to play the video game using only his or her brain waves. (This is actually easy; everyone can do it.) The specific brain wave frequencies are reinforced, and the sensor locations on the scalp are unique to each individual.

The professional observes the brain, via the EEG, assessing the test while in action. Neurofeedback refers to the process in which you learn to change your brainwaves and thus change the control of brain states. When other facilitators examine the brain activity via EEG, they can help the client change his or her brain activity by rewarding shifts toward a more functional and stable brain state.

Good self-regulation is necessary for optimal brain function. This training in self-regulating helps enhance the function of the central nervous system to improve mental performance, emotional control, and physiological stability.

Neurofeedback training has also been proven to improve attention. Neurofeedback can help to improve or eliminate anxiety, sleep problems, headaches, migraines, bedwetting, nightmares, stress reactions, depression, and emotional distress, as well as attention deficits and other forms of disruptive and disturbing behaviors. In addition, neurofeedback can help relieve traumatic brain injury, mood swings, and brain disorders such as seizures and strokes.

Neurofeedback does not "cure" conditions. It just helps the individual with self-regulating and improving his or her condition.

Social Skills Training

This training helps individuals with difficulties in socializing to develop and sustain meaningful and fulfilling peer relationships. People can exhibit inappropriate social behaviors for reasons ranging from neurological impairments to a lack of opportunity in acquiring these skills. Qualified therapists and psychologists teach appropriate socializing skills, such as initiating and maintaining positive social relationships with others. Difficulties with social skills generally include problems with reciprocity, initiating interactions and conversations, maintaining appropriate eye contact, enjoying appropriate fun experiences, understanding social cues, and understanding empathy.

One way to teach socialization is with social stories. These stories describe typical social situations, step by step, so that the child can understand what is expected of him or her in the social situation. Social skills are explained and taught in small groups via playing games, structured lesson plans, and role-playing activities. Having good matched peer groups is important.

Social skills training can help reduce anxiety and negative behaviors, keep the child from standing out as someone who is different, help prevent the child from being bullied, increase appropriate skills in a variety of social situations, and help increase self-confidence and self-esteem. The goal is not to change the uniqueness of the individual, but to improve skills and confidence, as they relate to the person's individual goals and aspirations.

Functional Behavioral Analysis

The first step in functional behavior analysis is having one or more trained professionals observe and describe the challenging behaviors that are interfering with a child's success at home, in school, or both. The professionals observe and track antecedents, behaviors, and consequences to understand the causes and the nature of the behavior. Baseline data collection is an important part of the assessment and helps professionals and parents track the effectiveness of recommended interventions and therapies. Interviewing the individual can provide insight into the child's perception of events at school or home.

The child could be displaying certain behaviors to gain attention, receive sensory stimuli, attempt to get a reward, attempt to self-regulate, escape from an uncomfortable situation or disliked activity, or fill a personal want or desire. Once an assessment has been completed, the examiner can refer the client to the appropriate professionals. They will develop and help parents implement a positive behavior support plan for home and school. To be successful, this therapy requires clear and consistent communication between parents and school officials.

Applied Behavior Analysis (ABA)

Applied behavior analysis teaches children social, motor, and verbal behaviors, as well as reasoning skills. ABA, also called behavior modification, works well with those who may not understand the cues of certain behaviors on their own, as typical children do. Parents, counselors, or certified behavior analysts can use the ABA approach. The emphasis is on rewarding appropriate behaviors.

Discrete Trial Teaching (DTT)

Discrete trial teaching or training helps children compensate for learning difficulties. DTT helps with limited attention spans by breaking down tasks into short, simple trials, taught one at a time. DTT also helps to build motivation by rewarding performance of desired behaviors and completion of tasks with tangible or external reinforcement, such as toys, food, or special privileges.

Children with ASDs often have difficulty understanding stimuli such as requests from an adult, communication from peers, or cues in the environment such as school bells, alarms, and different types of weather. The children are taught proper responses to the varieties of stimuli in their lives. This teaching technique or process is used to improve cognitive, communication, play, social, and self-help skills.

Pivotal Response Training (PRT)

Pivotal response treatment, or therapy, is a behavioral treatment intervention program, pioneered by Robert Koegel, PhD, and his wife, Lynn Koegel, PhD. The Koegels founded and run the Koegel Autism Research and Training Center at the University of California, Santa Barbara. PRT is based on the principles of ABA. It is child directed, while DTT is more therapist directed. With PRT, the child makes choices that direct the therapy. PRT uses reinforcements that are directly related to the task. The therapy focuses on treating language difficulties, as well as social, behavioral, and play deficits.

Relationship Development Intervention (RDI)

RDI was created by Steven Gutstein, PhD, and his wife, Rachelle Sheely, PhD. This parent-based intervention program addresses problems faced by children with ASD, such as learning about friendships, expressing empathy, and having a love of enjoying and sharing the world around them. The RDI approach trains and certifies clinicians to help parents implement an RDI program for their child. The program assists children with difficulties related to change of routine, and social and emotional development.

Eliminating Yeast

Many ASD children have an overgrowth of yeast in their intestines, mouth, and other areas. The GFCF diet helps eliminate many autistic traits, but removing yeast may help in making even more autistic traits vanish. Systemic yeast and imbalanced bacterial flora can cause a host of issues.

Fecal cultures, the urine tartaric acid test, and other lab tests can indicate an overgrowth of yeast, called Candida albicans. This overgrowth can cause hyperactivity, confusion, short attention span, lethargy, insomnia, irritability, and aggression, among other behaviors. Too much yeast also can cause health problems, such as headaches, stomachaches, constipation, gas pains, bloating, fatigue, and depression. If the tests prove that your child has an overgrowth of yeast, you can use medications to help eliminate it. Consult with your medical practitioner.

Candida albicans is a fungal organism that exists in everyone's intestinal tract. But when the balance is upset with an overgrowth, good bacteria can be destroyed. This often occurs because of antibiotic use or when the immune system is impaired by stress or illness. Candida can invade and colonize your body's tissues. Normally this organism is harmless, but an overgrowth can spread inside of the body and become a serious matter.

Ridding the body of excess yeast seems to help improve autistic children's sensory issues, eye contact, concentration, word usage, sleep patterns, imaginative play, academic performance, and appetite. It also can reduce hyperactive behaviors, repetitive behaviors such as spinning objects, eczema, rashes, and gut problems.

Foods that can cause yeast, and thus should be avoided, are those with simple sugars. These include white sugar, brown sugar, maple sugar, date sugar, raw sugar, turbinado, fruit juice, honey, molasses, maple syrup, corn syrup, and rice syrup, as well as many foods that you will avoid anyway because they contain gluten and casein.

Be aware, though, that some GFCF breads, rice, potatoes, and other starchy and sweet foods and cereals have a high glycemic index. This means they turn carbohydrates into sugars. These foods should also be avoided if yeast is an issue. For a list of foods with low, medium, and high glycemic indices, download the Glycemic Index PDF from the Canadian Diabetes Association website (http://www.diabetes.ca/for-professionals/resources/glycemic-index).

People with yeast issues sometimes prefer to use agave nectar as a sweetener and a healthy, natural sugar substitute, because it has a low glycemic index. Also, if yeast overgrowth is a problem, avoid foods containing vinegar, peanuts, mushrooms, and sorghum beans, as well as anything with the word "yeast" on the label.

Several fruits tend to be high in yeast and should be avoided. These are strawberries, grapes, raisins, dates, prunes, figs, other dried fruits, canned fruits, citrus, juices (home-squeezed are yeast free), and watermelon. Some teas should be avoided, as well as canned or prepared tomatoes (fresh are fine), parsnips, and jellybeans, which all have a high glycemic index. In addition, artificial sweeteners are to be avoided.

Only avoid these foods if your doctor or medical practitioner has found a yeast overgrowth and noted a problem. Your child will not need to eliminate these foods for life. Once the doctor sees that the gut is healed, he or she may give you permission to try the foods again while looking for a reaction or being tested for one.

Digestive Enzymes, Supplements, and Epsom Salt Bath Soaks

Some parents believe that giving their children enzymes will help counteract infractions when gluten or casein has been eaten accidentally. Many also feel that enzymes assist in digesting foods. Some parents also add dietary supplements to help improve ASD traits and behaviors. Medical practitioners have recommended trying various enzymes and supplements along with the GFCF diet. The websites listed here can provide background so that you can discuss enzymes and supplements with your child's health care provider.

Enzyme Stuff (http://www.enzymestuff.com/basicswhichenzyme.htm)
Autism Research Institute (http://www.autism.com/treatable/adams_biomed_summary.pdf)
Houston Enzymes (http://www.houstonni.com)
Kirkman Laboratories on enzymes (http://www.kirkmanlabs.com/products/enzymes/enzymes_index.html)
Kirkman Laboratories on multivitamins (http://www.kirkmanlabs.com/products/multivitamins/multivitamins_index.html)

Some brands or products that you might want to discuss with your child's medical practitioner to assist with viruses, yeast, phenols, or overall health are: Kirkman's Super Nu-Thera and Enzym-Complete; Houston's No-Fenol, Peptizyde, and Zyme Prime; and Enzymedica's Virastop, as well as amino acids, vitamin B12 with magnesium, antifungals, olive leaf extract, L-lysine, mB12, trimethylglycine, folic acid, carnitine, biotin, and grapefruit seed extract. Practitioners who've attended training sessions by Defeat Autism Now! often recommend these supplements and enzymes. Do your research and read everything you can about these products to see if they could help.

Another thing to try when an infraction occurs is an Epsom salt (magnesium sulfate) bath. Some people add baking soda to the water, as well. You will want to experiment with adding different amounts to the water. A common recommendation calls for one to two cups of Epsom salt in the bathwater. Once the Epsom salt and baking soda (or just the salt) has been added to the bathwater and dissolved, have your child sit and soak. Many parents say that this will remove the toxins.

Another bonus to using an Epsom salt soak is that it can extend your child's sleep cycle and ease digestive function. Epsom salt is readily available in most grocery stores and pharmacies, and even at home improvement centers. To learn more about Epsom salt, visit the Epsom Salt Council (http://www.epsomsaltcouncil.org).

B Vitamins

A lot has been said about how B vitamins can assist ASD children in improving many autistic traits. After taking B vitamins, many children have had impressive results with stimming, running out of control, eye contact, social skills, and behavior and language skills. Research B vitamins and speak to your doctor or medical practitioner about the benefits they might have for your child.

B-6 and B-12 are the B vitamins used most often to help children who have ASDs. Many doctors and medical practitioners who work with ASD children feel that they can benefit greatly by receiving extra B vitamins.

Vitamin B-12 is found in animal products such as meat, shellfish, milk, cheese, and eggs. Most people who eat these foods are not likely to develop a vitamin B-12 deficiency. Normally, there is enough vitamin B-12 stored in a person's liver to last a year, even if the person does not eat any foods that contain the vitamin during that time. Yet, because so many of our kids are picky eaters, they may not be getting enough B-12 even if they are following the GFCF Diet. Also, sometimes certain problems cause the body to not store B vitamins and they get flushed out.

To screen for B-12 deficiency, doctors and medical practitioners will ask for tests of serum and urine methylmalonic acid levels. However, many say that a child does not need to have low levels to benefit from B-12.

The vitamin is usually given via an intramuscular injection, but it also can be given in a nasal spray. Sometimes B-12 is given more frequently to start and then tapered off. For example, it might be given several times during the first week, then weekly for about three to six weeks, and then monthly for three months. Finally, the child is put on maintenance therapy. It works better when given with folic acid, which often is a deficiency for people with bowel disorders and epilepsy.

Vitamin B-12 does not work immediately. Improvement typically occurs two to four weeks after the first injection and lasts about four weeks. Some people report that three months can pass before improvements are seen with B-12.

B-6 is another vitamin used frequently to help children with ASD. Major sources of vitamin B-6 include: cereal grains, legumes, vegetables (carrots, spinach, peas), potatoes, milk, cheese, eggs, fish, liver, meat, and flour. Many of these foods are avoided on the GFCF Diet, so perhaps adding supplements makes sense. Vitamin B-6 can be found in pill form, chewable wafers, liquid, powdered, or a transdermal cream for the skin. An autistic person will only improve on a high dosage B-6 if his or her body requires extra B-6.

Benefits of B-6 often start within a few days. If no benefits are seen in three to four weeks (which occurs in about 50 percent of the cases), or if any signs of peripheral neuropathy appear (which is very rare), you should stop giving the B-6. Vitamin B-6 is recommended for use in conjunction with magnesium.

Taken orally, the B vitamins are among the worst tasting ingredients in vitamin and mineral supplements. A transdermal B-complex cream is available that contains B-1, B-2 (riboflavin), B-3, B-5, B-6 (P-5-P), biotin, and optionally folinic acid. The drawback is that the riboflavin temporarily colors the skin orange. The color disappears over several hours and can be washed off clothing easily.

For parents that have difficulties with the orange color in the transdermal B-complex cream, a colorless version is available through some sources. The colorless cream does not contain riboflavin, but there are other ways to get riboflavin into the system.

Being Concerned with Phenols and Salicylates

Phenols and salicylates may sound like odd words, or perhaps they are just words that you never heard before. But by being knowledgeable about phenols and salicylates, you may be able to make an even greater difference in your child's health, behavior, and all-around well-being. First, let us discuss what phenols and salicylates are and where they exist in our diets.

Salicylates are natural chemicals made by many plants and are a subset of phenols. Salicylates are chemically related to aspirin, which is a derivative of salicylic acid. It is believed that the plant uses it as protection from insects. Although natural salicylates are found in wholesome foods, some individuals have difficulty tolerating even small amounts of them. If a person is highly sensitive, the reaction to a natural salicylate can be as severe as that to synthetic additives. Some people experience problems with only one or two, while others are sensitive to many or all of them.

Here are symptoms that may appear when children have reactions to phenols or salicylates, or both:
- Dark circles under the eyes
- Red face and ears
- Diarrhea

- Hyperactivity
- Impulsivity
- Aggression
- Headache
- Head banging or other self-injury
- Inappropriate laughter
- Impatience
- Short attention span
- Difficulty falling asleep at night
- Hives
- Stomachaches
- Bed-wetting and day wetting
- Dyslexia
- Speech difficulties
- Tics
- Some forms of seizures
- Night waking for several hours

Some people say they have seen improvements in the traits listed above by removing some or all of the following foods from their child's diet:

- Apples
- Grapes
- Oranges
- Peppers
- Berries
- Tomatoes
- Chocolate or cocoa
- Peanuts
- Bananas

Additives and salicylates are a primary concern for the Feingold Association, named after Benjamin Feingold, MD. He developed a diet free of artificial additives and some salicylates to treat or reduce behaviors of ADHD. Its use has been expanded to other groups, such as ASD children. (The Feingold Diet will be discussed in more detail later in this chapter.)

While the association's primary emphasis is on food, the group also recommends avoiding non-food products that could be potentially troublesome. Salicylates can be found in:

- Toiletries
- Sunscreens
- Cleaning supplies
- Art supplies containing synthetic or artificial colors and flavors (for example, FD&C colors, vanillin) or petroleum-based preservatives such as BHA, BHT, and TBHQ.
- Some natural flavorings and colorings that may include aspirin, and products containing aspirin or salicylic acid.

The Feingold Diet suggests avoiding foods at first that could produce adverse reactions, as stated above. These foods are listed in alphabetical order:

- Almonds
- Apples (juice, fruit, sauce)
- Apricots
- Berries (all)
- Cherries
- Chili powder
- Cider vinegar and apple cider
- Cloves
- Coffee
- Cucumbers and pickles

- Currants
- Grapes
- Nectarines
- Oranges
- Paprika
- Peaches
- Peppers (bell and chili)
- Plums
- Prunes
- Raisins
- Tangerines
- Tea
- Tomatoes
- Wine vinegar and wine
- Oil of wintergreen (methyl salicylate)
- Rosehips

The following additives are not routinely eliminated on the Feingold Diet, but many families prefer to avoid them. The Feingold Association designates the presence of these additives in foods to make the symptoms they may cause easier to identify.

- Nitrites and nitrates
- Corn sweeteners
- Monosodium glutamate and hydrolyzed vegetable protein
- Sulfiting agents
- Sodium benzoate
- Calcium propionate
- Natural smoke flavoring

Feingold *Foodlists* are books listing thousands of acceptable brand-name foods, tailored for each region of the United States. The first 100-plus pages of each *Foodlist* are devoted to acceptable nonsalicylate foods and non-food products. The rest of the book contains lists of acceptable brand-name products that contain one or more of the salicylates.

You probably will not need to eliminate *all* of these products. But, as stated in Chapter 1, at least get rid of anything artificial. Next eliminate all of the above-mentioned products temporarily, and then add one each week, keeping track in your diary as you look for symptoms to appear. If you see no changes after a week, or even after three or so days, take that food away, add another food, and look for symptoms. Continue to do this with all of the foods on the list.

Some items might cause reactions within a few hours or a day or two. Keep track, paying attention to which foods show reactions and how soon they appear. You then might want to try similar foods to see if they cause the same reaction, continuing until the list has been completed. Again, remove the problem-causing foods first, so you are not confused by what was causing the behavior.

The Feingold materials describe how to reintroduce salicylates and identify the reactions that these foods might cause.

Be Informed about Other Allergens and Intolerances

As stated previously, the top six allergens (not counting milk and wheat) are soy, shellfish, fish, eggs, peanuts, and tree nuts. Investigate if any of them cause your child to be intolerant or to exhibit allergic reactions. You should also consider other common allergens, such as corn, rice, and potatoes.

You will not know if your child has issues with these foods unless you eliminate them and reintroduce them into his or her diet, or if he or she tested positive to them in an allergy test. Eliminating these items will give you even more practice in reading labels. Seeing if your child will react inappropriately to these allergens is all trial and error.

Chelation

Many parents of ASD children have heard of chelation (pronounced key-LAY-shun), but they might not know exactly what is involved. In chelation, a chemical substance is used to remove toxins from the body orally, intravenously, or transdermally (by rubbing cream or gel onto the skin). The chelating chemicals are introduced into the body to bind metals or minerals, such as lead, mercury, and cadmium, into molecules. Chelation has been scientifically proven to remove excess or toxic metals before they can cause damage to the body.

However, chelation should only be done if your doctor or healthcare practitioner prescribes it. The doctor should have your child tested for heavy metal toxicity to see if this procedure is warranted before you start. Learn the risks and the benefits, and decide whether or not to try this method based on your thoughts and those of your medical practitioner. To find out more about chelation, you might want to start reading these message boards for answers or to ask some questions of your own: Yahoo Groups' Autism-Mercury group (http://health.groups.yahoo. com/group/Autism-Mercury) or ChelatingKids2 group (http://health. groups.yahoo.com/group/chelatingkids2).

Hyperbaric Oxygen Therapy

Most people have heard of a hyperbaric chamber being used to cure the bends for deep-sea divers who have surfaced too quickly. Hyperbaric oxygen therapy (HBOT) has recently been used to help ASD children. The hyperbaric chamber is a pressurized enclosure with higher-than-normal atmospheric pressure. HBOT treatments seem to help increase cerebral blood flow, delivering oxygen to areas of the brain that are thought to be oxygen deficient.

HBOT has been found to aid in the recovery of idling neurons because greater amounts of blood and oxygen stimulate the cerebral tissues. HBOT also helps reduce excess fluids and the swelling of the brain tissues, which improves neurological function for those with ASDs and makes them less confused.

In addition, HBOT can assist in the removal of heavy metals, such as mercury. Sometimes HBOT and chelation can be done simultaneously, or one after the other, for maximum benefits in removing toxic metals. Scans are usually completed before and after HBOT sessions to compare results. Many parents have reported that after HBOT treatments, their child has had increased language and improved social skills.

Other Diets to Investigate

Besides the GFCF Diet, many parents choose to investigate other diet options that might help their child, in addition to being on the GFCF Diet. Here is information on several of the more popular approaches for ASD kids. Some people choose to combine the GFCF and one or more of these diets. They might be worth considering.

The Feingold Diet

The Feingold Diet (http://www.feingold.org), which I have mentioned several times already in this book, has helped many children with problems such as:

- Hyperactive behavior
- Short attention span
- Disruptive behavior
- Unresponsiveness to discipline
- Unkindness to pets
- Poor self-control and destructive behaviors, such as throwing or breaking things
- Little or no recognition of danger to self
- Inappropriate noises
- Excessive talking
- Loud talking

- Interrupting often
- Abusive behavior
- Unpredictable behavior
- Aggression
- Perseveration or repetition of an activity
- Touching things or people excessively
- Workaholic habits
- Chewing on clothing or other objects
- Scratching, biting, and picking at the skin
- Low tolerance for frustration
- Depression or frequent crying
- Demanding immediate attention
- Irritability
- Overreaction to touch, pain, sound, or lights
- Panicking easily or nervousness
- Low self-esteem
- Mood swings
- Suicidal thoughts
- Tendency to be accident prone
- Poor muscle coordination
- Difficulty writing and drawing
- Dyslexia and reading problems
- Speech difficulties or delays
- Difficulty with playground activities and sports
- Eye muscle disorder (nystagmus, strabismus)
- Tics (unusual or uncontrollable movements)
- Auditory memory deficits (difficulty remembering what is heard)
- Visual memory deficits (difficulty remembering what is seen)
- Difficulty in comprehension and short-term memory
- Disturbance in spatial orientation (up-down, right-left)
- Difficulties in reasoning (simple math problems, meaning in words)

- Sleep problems
- Ear infections
- Asthma
- Bed-wetting (enuresis)
- Daytime wetting
- Stomachaches
- Headaches and migraines
- Hives and rashes (urticaria)
- Eczema
- Leg aches
- Constipation
- Diarrhea
- Congestion
- Seizures (especially if combined with migraines or hyperactivity)

Benjamin Feingold, MD, who passed away in 1982, was a pediatrician, allergist, and Chief of Allergy at Kaiser Permanente Medical Center in San Francisco. In his practice, he noticed that some of his patients reacted to particular foods and food additives. He found, to his surprise, that while some people had physical reactions, many also experienced changes in their behavior. Many people are aware that alcohol, nicotine, caffeine, and drugs can affect behavior. But, most people do not realize that chemicals added to foods may also do serious harm.

In the late 1960s and early 1970s, Dr. Feingold developed what he called the "K-P" diet (for Kaiser Permanente). The diet was based on the Lockey Allergy Diet used at the Mayo Clinic.

Using the diet as originally designed, Dr. Feingold found that he could help about half of the children diagnosed with what was then called hyperkinesis, but now is called ADHD. When he refined the diet to remove the preservatives BHA and BHT, the success rate increased to about 70 percent. The media changed the name of the K-P diet to the Feingold Diet.

There are two parts to the Feingold Diet. During Stage One, additives, preservatives, and salicylates are removed from the person's diet and lifestyle. You must remove all artificial colors (dyes); artificial flavors; the preservatives BHA, BHT, and TBHQ; aspartame (known as NutraSweet or Equal); all natural salicylates, in any form; and anything containing aspirin in food and non-food items.

Stage Two follows, if Stage One has been successful. During Stage Two, salicylate foods are reintroduced, one by one, while the person is watched for negative reactions. (Note: Do not ever reintroduce the artificial additives and chemicals.) If you are doing this, keep a diary to help you be aware of behaviors, sensory issues, health issues, or attitudes that you see, both positive and negative.

Try one of the salicylates on the list for about week, charting any reactions that you see. Provide the freshest foods, if possible. If you see negative responses, stop giving that food immediately. Keep track of which foods cause which reaction or improvement. Then, during the next week, try another salicylate food, again watching for a reaction, good or bad. Continue this until all of the foods have been tried.

Keep in mind that different forms of fruit (dried, raw, cooked, or juice) may elicit different responses. If a person cannot tolerate fresh apples, for example, do not give up on all apple products. Apple juice might still be okay.

Different varieties of fruits might also have different effects. A child may do fine with a green apple, but not with a red or yellow one. The same is true for varieties of grapes. Sensitivity can change through the years, so you might want to reintroduce some of the foods again later to observe if a reaction appears.

The nonprofit Feingold Association of the United States was founded by parents in 1976. The association is run mostly by volunteers who have seen the value of the Feingold Diet. The association performs detailed research into food products, including fast food, as well as store-bought and non-food products, such as cosmetics and hygiene products. The association newsletter, called *Pure Facts*, comes out ten times a year and is full of facts, information, and data. Through emails and the newsletter, the association keeps families posted on any changes in ingredients or other important information.

The association also offers several books on how to follow the diet that list thousands of products available in most grocery stores and specialty stores which are acceptable to purchase. Member materials include suggested meal plans and recipes; information on finding acceptable supplements and medicine; and a detailed guide to many fast-food chains.

Volunteers at the Feingold Association are available to assist anyone who calls with a problem or question and to help figure out why symptoms are not improving.

Results can appear within three days with the diet, or they make take as long as three weeks. Everything must be changed, as stated previously. Even one bite of a food with an artificial dye could set your child up for failure. Infractions can occur in many ways, just like with the GFCF Diet. Although people may not be aware of these infractions, they can be potentially risky.

Keeping a diary is the only way infractions will be recognizable. The problem could be as simple as dye in a medication that the child has taken. The Feingold Association warns parents that although a food is labeled, "No preservatives," it may still contain them. The product, for example, could have been made in oil that contained preservatives. The Feingold manuals help answer some of these questions.

The Body Ecology Diet

The Body Ecology Diet (BED; http://www.bodyecologydiet.com) was developed by Donna Gates, a nutritional consultant, to help reverse fungal infections including candidiasis. This infection occurs when there is an overgrowth of the yeast or fungus known as Candida.

The first step in the diet is introducing young coconut kefir to help heal the gut. Kefir is a natural probiotic. It contains live, active cultures of normal flora that can help the digestive tract and aid in digestion. Young coconut kefir is made from young coconuts, sometimes referred to as green coconuts. This is not to be confused with coconut "milk," which is from mature coconuts. Nutritionally, mature coconut "milk" is not the same as juice or liquid from a young coconut.

Most areas of the United States sell these coconuts, which are often imported from Thailand. The coconuts are shaved down and just the white husk is packaged for sale. If the coconuts are not available, you can search for young green coconut water. Both the water and juice from inside the young coconut need to be fermented before being consumed as a beverage or yogurt.

The coconut juice is fermented for eighteen to forty-eight hours, using a kefir starter. (Time varies due to many factors.) Young coconut kefir is loaded with vitamin C, vitamin B, phosphorus, amino acids, enzymes, calcium, and magnesium. For help in making your young coconut kefir, visit the Kefir website (http://www.kefir.net). Check with your health-food store to purchase kefir starter or search for it online.

The second food to be added on the BED is raw butter. Raw butter is said to be 99 percent casein free. Some parents who have adapted the GFCF Diet and wish to remain GFCF have been concerned about the casein in raw butter. The Donna Gates' staff found that if the butter was introduced four to seven days after the young coconut kefir, the casein did not cause problems. Some children who react to even the slightest amount of casein may have problems eating raw butter.

Another aspect of the BED is eating foods that are natural, such as vegetables, "meats" (chicken, turkey, lamb and fish), free-range eggs, and good fats, and using Celtic sea salt and herbs for seasoning. The BED recommends using gluten-free grains, such as millet, buckwheat, amaranth, and quinoa. These grains help alkalinize the body, which is another goal of the BED.

The BED also recommends using fatty acids such as antifungal and antiviral coconut oil, vitamins A and D, cod liver oil or krill oil, unrefined seed oils like pumpkin-seed oil (zinc), flaxseed oil (omega 3), borage (gamma-linolenic acid and omega 6), evening primrose, and casein-free ghee. Green juice made from broccoli stems, a leafy green, and celery is also recommended. You can also add an avocado to a juicer to make this juice.

For more information on this diet, read Donna Gates's book, called *The Body Ecology Diet*.

Sara's Diet

Sara's Diet is not as well known as some of the other diets, but I have included it because some children have had success with it.

The diet was investigated and introduced by Max and Sandra Desorgher, formerly Sandra Johnson, and was named after Sandra's daughter, Sara. A key component of Sara's Diet is eliminating foods with lutein. Foods highest in lutein are kale, spinach, mustard greens, yellow corn, broccoli, green peas, pumpkin, collard greens, summer (yellow) squash, carrots, brussels sprouts, red currants, green olives, peppers (green, orange, and yellow), green beans (pod), chicken fat, egg yolk, plums, peaches, oranges, tangerines, avocados, kiwi, and rhubarb. Lutein often is also contained in the peel of fruits and vegetables such as cucumbers, pears, and pineapples. The dark outer leaves of cabbage, lettuce, and leeks contain lutein, and strawberries contain a red form called vitellorubin.

Sara's Diet also requires eliminating artificial food dyes and the artificial sweetener aspartame. The diet might also include removing or reducing the intake of gluten or casein, or both, as well as soy protein, other carotene pigments, and high purine foods (sweetbreads, anchovies, sardines, liver, beef kidneys, brains, meat extracts (such as Oxo or Bovril), herring, mackerel, scallops, game meats, and gravy).

In addition, followers of this diet may remove active dry yeast, monosodium glutamate, and excessive supplements. They also may return to some dairy fats and grains that were unnecessarily removed, in the opinion of those promoting this diet.

Withdrawal symptoms may occur during the first four months of this diet. To avoid reactions to the changes in the body, those promoting this diet suggest adding B-vitamins, honey, dimethylglycine, coenzyme Q10, and cod-liver oil.

If you are interested in investigating this diet more, visit the World Community Autism Program website (http://www.saras-autism-diet. freeservers.com/Diet/Saras_Diet_I.html) and discuss its contents with your medical practitioner.

The Specific Carbohydrate Diet

The Specific Carbohydrate Diet (SCD) assists the digestive system by eliminating grains and many sugars from the diet. Elaine Gottschall knew she had to do something because her daughter was unable to keep any food down. She got sicker and sicker. Most of the doctors that saw her were of no help.

Elaine, her husband, and their daughter finally met a doctor who asked about the food their daughter was eating. He was the first doctor to mention "the food." After listening to him, Elaine and her husband changed their daughter's diet. She began eating mostly meats, fruits, and vegetables and eliminated carbohydrates such as grains, flour, and sugar. Before their eyes, Elaine and her husband saw their daughter recover from her severe intestinal and neurological disorders.

Elaine decided she had to save other children and continue the legacy of the doctor who had saved her daughter's life. At age forty-seven, Elaine returned to school to become a biochemist and write the book *Breaking the Vicious Cycle*. This book has sold more than one million copies and is available in twelve languages. Although Elaine passed away in 2005, her book has helped many people who suffer from Crohn's disease, ulcerative colitis, irritable bowel syndrome, celiac disease, diverticulitis, autism, cystic fibrosis, and other ailments rooted in the digestive tract.

The foods that need to be avoided on the SCD are sugars with double molecules (disaccharides such as lactose, sucrose, maltose, and isomaltose) and starches (polysaccharides). The starches in all grains, corn, and potatoes must also be strictly avoided. Corn syrup is also excluded because it contains a mixture of short-chain starches.

Some legumes, dried beans, lentils, and split peas, which are forms of starches, have been tolerated. However, you must soak them for ten to twelve hours before cooking them. Discard the soaking water because it contains other indigestible sugars that are removed in the soaking process. Small amounts of legumes may be added to the diet after about three months to see if they can be tolerated.

Homemade fermented yogurt is allowed on the SCD, but not on the GFCF Diet. The yogurt helps heal the gut by increasing the good bacteria. The yogurt must be fermented for at least twenty-four hours. Store-bought yogurt is not allowed. Other than this homemade yogurt, no dairy products are allowed on the SCD.

Some people who have been on the GFCF Diet say that their ASD children have tolerated this special recipe for fermented yogurt, when made with goat milk and when specifically following the SCD recipe. (Normally goat milk is not allowed on the GFCF Diet.)

For more information on this yogurt, go to the Kids & SCD website (http://www.pecanbread.com/new/yogurt1.html). You can find more about the diet and how it has helped ASD children at the same website (http://www.pecanbread.com). For information about additional foods that are allowed and disallowed on the SCD, go to the website for *Breaking the Vicious Cycle* (http://www.breakingtheviciouscycle.info/legal/legal_illegal_a-c.htm).

Chapter 14

⫸ Spreading the Word ⫷

I have initiated the crusade of speaking to families all over the world about the beneficial GFCF Diet for children with ASD and those with other disorders.

I sit on several advocacy boards, one through *The Autism Perspective* magazine, for which I wrote an article about the GFCF Diet in spring 2006, and another through the Autism Network for Dietary Intervention (http://www.autismndi.com).

This diet has been proven time and again to help children and adults with autism, Asperger syndrome, pervasive developmental disorder, attention deficit disorder with and without hyperactivity, sensory integration dysfunction, oppositional defiant disorder, and even Down syndrome. This message must be heard by the parents of children with these conditions and disorders.

After implementing this diet for my son, I knew my calling was to "pay it forward" to thousands of parents the world over to bring a change to their lives, so that they, too, could experience the miracle that we see every day.

My crusade got under way with a few published articles. Besides the article for *The Autism Perspective*, I wrote an article for the Autism Society of America's newsletter, one for a newspaper called *The Acorn*, one for Arico Foods, and one for *Living Without* magazine (June–July 2008). I continue to write articles about this important topic, most recently contributing to *Fresno Magazine*'s Medical Guide for 2009.

I realized that my message, my mission, and my passion needed to reach thousands of other parents around the world. I then decided that I had to write this book, to further inform parents that changes can be accomplished safely that will improve their child's behavior and help with their child's overall well-being. These changes will improve not just their child's life, but those of everyone around them.

I started to speak at local support groups, sharing my knowledge and offering follow-up help to parents who needed support. I realized if I could walk parents through Whole Foods Market and Trader Joe's and give them tours, they could see all of the GFCF foods in the stores that they might have overlooked.

On its website, Trader Joe's has a list of the GF foods (http://traderjoes.com/Attachments/NoGluten.pdf) and vegan (casein-free and egg-free) foods (http://traderjoes.com/Attachments/Vegan.pdf) that the company sells. (Realize that the gluten-free and vegan foods are listed separately, and you will have to verify that any item is free of other foods that you need to avoid.)

Whole Foods Market came out with a list of the stores' GFCF foods in 2008. You can find the information and print it out from the Whole Foods website (http://www.wholefoodsmarket.com/specialdiets). Many Whole Foods stores have copies at their facilities, too. Whole Foods also offers separate lists of just gluten free and just dairy free for those not doing both at the same time.

The tours have been very successful in helping parents locate many foods that they might not find on their own. Being familiar with the store helps tremendously, especially if they had not shopped there much before. Thousands of new GFCF products are showing up on the shelves daily as manufacturers become aware of the need for more of these foods. If you shop often, you will see the new items. If you do not shop frequently enough, you will not be aware of the many new foods that are beginning to adorn the shelves.

If you become skilled with this diet and wish to give back, I urge you to volunteer to give tours at your local health-food store, Whole Foods Market, Trader Joe's, or whichever stores in your community offer the most GFCF products. In smaller towns, where no major natural, healthy grocery stores exist, perhaps a tour of the regular grocery store is more in order. Pointing out the specialty items on such a tour would be very beneficial.

Look around your community for online support groups through which you can email information to parents about your tours. Check with local support groups, autism societies, and special needs groups through your school district, agencies that assist children with special needs, speech pathologists, ABA providers, behaviorists, and physicians. Of course, one of the best ways is just networking by word of mouth.

Become an expert and offer your services to other parents who will be ever so grateful. If you live in an area without support groups and services, it might be time to start your own network. With one out of 150 children being diagnosed with ASDs, you are sure to find other parents seeking support.

One way to gather individuals is to start a meet-up group. These groups are all over the world and can pertain to any subject. Before you start a group, see if an autism, ADHD, or GFCF group is already set up in or near your community. If not, you can start one at Meetup Inc.'s website (http://www.meetup.com).

Put an ad in the newspaper, on bulletin boards at parks, and at religious establishments, schools, or other locations where parents will see it. You may want to write a letter to the editor in a local newspaper inviting parents to a support group. Churches and synagogues often will offer you a room free of charge where you can hold your meetings. Call around to find a free room, or use someone's living room to hold your meetings. Talk about the GFCF Diet and autism, and offer to arrange tours.

Spread the word!

Chapter 15

⫸ My Son Noah's Story... ⫷
In His Own Words

I am now twelve years old. I was diagnosed with autism at age six. When I was seven years old, my mom started me on the GFCF Diet.

I have no recollection of my autistic past, but my mom remembers well. According to her, I would have horrendous meltdowns, and I was mean or hurtful to other children. I could not go outside without sunglasses, and loud noises "freaked me out."

Nobody with the right mind likes garlic, and I am no exception, for if I was within the same room as such or onions, I would refuse to show my face and immediately got the heck out of there. My meals solely consisted of peanut butter and jelly sandwiches on wheat bread, yogurt, massive quantities of milk, ice cream, cottage cheese, and other food items that are now simply unholy.

My mother thought I would starve when she heard about the diet. Once I was on the diet, however, an amazing aura of light came upon me. I now enjoy eating a variety of foods, including meat and chicken. Before the diet, meat was like the devil's horse hockey. Now, it is like a gift from above.

I can now eat out at certain places (very, *very* rarely getting the entire meal), such as an occasional visit to In-N-Out (no sauces, dressings, or bun on the burger should be the only change; the french fries are legal, and so is 7UP). P.F. Chang's is one of my favorite places to eat; they actually have a gluten-free menu. P.F. Chang's does not have a menu that is both gluten and dairy free, but, coincidentally, the only item on the gluten-free menu that has dairy is the cake.

One of my other favorite restaurants is Storytellers Café at Disney's Grand Californian Hotel. Storytellers Café does not have dedicated GFCF menus—but the chef there is more than willing to accommodate your requests. (Almost all of Disney's eateries can accommodate special diets.)

Another positive effect of the diet is that my grades in school have skyrocketed. Before the diet, my grades were A's, B's, and C's, and my behavior could grant me no higher than an S for citizenship and work habits. (My school's grades are as follows: U for unsatisfactory, the worst possible; N for needs improvement; S for satisfactory; and E for excellent, the best possible.)

Two years ago, in my first year of middle school (after four years of the diet), my first-trimester report card sported straight A's and E's. That was, needless to say, one of my best accomplishments—because of it, I got my first Nintendo DS handheld video game system. (☺) As of this writing, I have just completed my seventh grade year with all honors classes (which is to say honors math, English, and social studies—my school does not have seventh grade honors science for some reason).

Naturally, those honors classes are extremely tough; I am now back to mostly A's, very few B's, mostly E's, and a few S's. (The only reason I have S's is because of one particular teacher who must be against people with disabilities. All of my other teachers were willing to accommodate my minor needs, whereas I seemed to annoy this one. He still gave me an A in the class.)

My social status is actually low because I do not share the same interests as the majority of other kids; I am not into boy-girl relationships, life-scarring M-rated video games, and television shows that kids my age should not be watching, so half of it is an adolescent problem. In fact, it is sometimes hard to differentiate whether it has to do with such or autism.

Aside from all of these differences, however, I am an overall normal, albeit somewhat shy, boy. I am not teased because of these differences (to my knowledge); on the contrary, the majority of students seem to praise them, or at least the most apparent one—a severe impairment to my handwriting neatness, which forces me to use what I call an "AlphaSmart" (the "assistive device" mentioned in the first chapter of this book). Everybody seems to think that it is "cool" to type everything, which, after all these years, has lost its flair to me.

Overall, my life, after many years and with some accommodations, has become normal. There are many people I would like to thank for this:

First of all, my parents, who, despite their divorce, have (mostly) worked together to help me on my travels through life. Second, my therapists, who have helped me just as much, if not more, on that journey. Third, most (remember that "S" guy I mentioned earlier?) of my teachers, for without their understanding and willingness to accommodate, I would be an entirely different person. I would like to name them all, but there are simply too many of them. And lastly, all of my pets over the years. To them, I can only say that you have my undying gratitude.

✒ Resources ✒

Stores That Carry GFCF Foods
To find an organic food store near you:

http://www.organicstorelocator.com

http://www.domatalivingflour.com/ordergfcfflourhere

http://www.sylvanborderfarm.com

http://www.madwomanfoods.com/commercecgi/commerce.
   cgi?page=Terms.htm

http://auntcandicefoods.com

http://www.naturesflavors.com

http://www.glutenfreeoats.com

http://www.glutenfreeflour.com

http://www.glutenfreecreations.com

http://www.glutenfreebagelcompany.com

http://www.123glutenfree.com

http://thecravingsplace.com

http://www.gfessentials.com

http://www.wheatfreefood.com

http://www.glutenfree-supermarket.com

http://www.glutenevolution.com

http://www.curiouscookie.com/cookies/glutenfree.asp
http://www.glutenfreebcg.com/default.php
http://www.grindstonebakery.com
http://www.cravebakery.org
http://www.newcascadiatraditional.com
http://www.rheinlanderbakery.com
http://www.sprouts.com
http://www.localharvest.org
http://www.glutenfreepizza.com
http://www.glutenfreeforme.com/index.htm
http://www.glutensmart.com
http://www.gfsoap.com
http://www.galaxyfoods.com
http://www.gilliansfoods.com
http://www.sunnybridgenaturalfoods.com
http://www.thegrainlessbaker.com
http://www.glutenfreefabulous.com

Eating Outside the USA

Purchasing Food, Ordering Food, and Restaurant Listings

Here's a great site to help with gluten-free international travel, or for those living in countries outside of the United States: Celiac Travel (http://www.celiactravel.com). Note that this information is only gluten free.

If a website is in a language that you do not understand, use these websites for free to translate words into the language that you understand best:

http://babelfish.altavista.com
http://translation2.paralink.com
http://www.freetranslation.com
http://www.google.com/translate_t

By Country

Some countries' celiac/coeliac societies and support groups are listed below by country name to provide you with additional, helpful information.

Make sure that the foods are both gluten free and casein free, as well as any other allergens or intolerances that you must avoid.

Here is a site listing health-food stores and co-ops in many parts of the world: http://www.organicconsumers.org/foodcoops.htm

Argentina
http://www.geocities.com/acelanqn
http://www.celiaco.org.ar/uk.asp
http://www.celiachandbook.com/argentina.html

Australia
http://www.coeliac.org.au
http://wa.coeliacsociety.com.au
http://sa.coeliacsociety.com.au
http://www.nswcoeliac.org.au
http://www.glutenfreeshop.com.au/front.htm
http://www.glutenfreefavourites.com.au
http://www.glutenfreewarehouse.com.au
http://www.onlyoz.com.au
http://www.yourrestaurants.com.au
http://www.celiachandbook.com/australia.html
http://www.anzwers.org/free/gfcf/shopping.html
http://santostrading.com.au
http://www.alfalfahouse.org
http://www.wagamama.com.au

Austria
http://www.zoeliakie.or.at

Belgium

http://vcv.coeliakie.be/tiki-index.php
http://www.wagamama.be

Bermuda

http://www.rockonforhealth.com

Brazil

http://www.acelbra.org.br/english/index.php
http://www.semgluten.com.br

Canada

http://www.celiac.ca
http://www.celiachandbook.com/canada.html
https://www.sickkids.on.ca/sfs_site/shopping/customerservice.asp
http://www.penny.ca/Stores.htm
http://www.planetorganic.ca
http://www.superstore.ca
http://www.bulkbarnfoods.com
http://www.happycow.net/north_america/canada
http://www.amaranthfoods.ca (Alberta)
http://www.communitynaturalfoods.com (Alberta)
http://www.celiac.edmonton.ab.ca/sources.html (Alberta)
http://www.glutenfreeisthewaytobe.com (British Columbia)
http://www.capersmarkets.com (British Columbia)
http://www.stongs.com/index.cfm?fuseaction=content&c_id=6 (British
   Columbia)
http://www.organzamarket.com (Manitoba)
http://www.celiac.ottawa.on.ca/suppliers.htm#suppliers (Ontario)
http://www.naturesemporium.ca (Ontario)
http://www.onfc.ca (Ontario)

http://www.elpeto.com/outletstore.html (Ontario)
http://www.ecollegey.com (Quebec)
http://www.casagranby.com/english/casa.html (Quebec)
http://eathealthyfoods.ca (Saskatchewan)

China
http://www.celiachandbook.com/china.html

Croatia
http://www.celijakija.hr

Czech Republic
http://www.coeliac.cz/en
http://www.celiac.cz
http://www.celiachandbook.com/czech.html

Denmark
http://www.coeliaki.dk
http://www.madtildig.dk

Finland
http://www.keliakialiitto.fi
http://www.allermiina.fi/shop
http://www.celiachandbook.com/finland.html

France
http://www.afdiag.org
http://www.celiachandbook.com/france.html
http://www.sansglutensanscaseine.com
http://www.labelviesansgluten.com
http://www.valpiform.net

http://www.natama.fr
http://www.lavieclaire.com
http://www.naturalia.fr
http://www.biosphare.com
http://www.dietetiquemouffetard.fr/index.htm?lang=en
http://www.glutabye.com
http://www.lereminet.com

Germany

http://www.celiachandbook.com/germany.html
http://www.dzg-online.de
http://www.schaer.com
http://www.zoeliakie-net.de
http://www.glutenfrei-lebenswelt.de

Holland (See Netherlands)

Hungary

http://www.celiachandbook.com/hungary.html
http://www.coeliac.hu

India

http://www.celiacsocietyindia.com
http://nutritionfoundationofindia.res.in

Ireland

http://www.coeliac.ie/food.htm
http://www.celiachandbook.com/ireland.html
http://www.wagamama.ie
http://www.giulianipharma.ie/index.htm

Israel
http://www.celiac.org.il
http://www.GlutenFree.co.il ("English"tab in the upper left corner, if needed)

Italy
http://www.celiachandbook.com/italy.html
http://www.celiachia.it/ristoratori/default_eng.asp
http://prodottibiologici.it

Luxembourg
http://www.alig.lu

Netherlands
http://www.coeliakievereniging.nl
http://www.celiachandbook.com/netherlands.html
http://www.glutenvrij-lepoole.nl/site.php
http://www.glutenfree.nl
http://www.glutenvrijemarkt.com
http://www.glutenvrijewebshop.nl
http://www.gluten-vrij.nl
http://www.ekoplaza.nl
http://www.wagamama.nl

Norway
http://www.celiachandbook.com/norway.html
http://www.ncf.no
http://www.glutenfri.org

New Zealand
http://colourcards.com/coeliac
http://www.glutenfreegoodies.co.nz

http://www.ieproduce.com
http://www.wagamama.co.nz

Philippines
http://www.freelivingfoods.com/index.htm

Poland
http://www.bezgluten.pologne.pl/oferta.php

Portugal
http://www.celiacos.org.pt

Puerto Rico
http://www.freshmartpr.com

Romania
http://celiachie.uniserve.ro

Scotland
http://www.grassrootsorganic.com

Singapore
http://www.organic-paradise.com.sg
http://www.natures-glory.com/home.asp
http://www.supernature.com.sg/index.php
http://sg.geocities.com/roycelim2001/HFS.htm
http://www.coldstorage.com.sg/mall (Great World City)
http://www.theconsciouschoice.com/cake/contact.htm

South Africa
http://www.o-crumbs.com

http://www.earthmother.co.za
http://www.celiachandbook.com/southafrica.html
http://www.restaurants.co.za
http://www.refreshcafe.co.za
http://www.knet.co.za/healthfood/manufact.htm
http://www.showcook.co.za/Organics.htm

Spain

http://www.celiacscatalunya.org
http://www.celiacosmadrid.org/actualidad_19.html
http://www.celiachandbook.com/spain.html

Sweden

http://www.celiaki.se
http://www.celiachandbook.com/sweden.html

Switzerland

http://www.zoeliakie.ch
http://www.gfshop.ch
http://www.reformhaus.ch

Turkey

http://www.colyak.web.tr

UK

http://www.coeliac.co.uk
http://www.glutenfree-foods.co.uk
http://www.gffdirect.co.uk
http://www.celiachandbook.com/uk.html
http://www.theglutenfreekitchen.co.uk
http://www.goodfooddelivery.co.uk

http://www.gfree.co.uk
http://www.intolerablefood.com
http://www.sainsburys.co.uk/home.htm
http://www.goodnessdirect.co.uk
http://www.dietaryneedsdirect.co.uk
http://www.latasca.co.uk
http://www.eat.co.uk/pages/facts.html

Uruguay
http://www.acelu.org

Virgin Islands
http://www.naturesway.vg

Message Boards/ListServs/Forums on Diets, Interventions, and ASD

http://health.groups.yahoo.com/group/GFCFKids
http://health.groups.yahoo.com/group/Autism_in_Girls
http://health.groups.yahoo.com/group/Autism_LDN
http://health.groups.yahoo.com/group/autism-aspergers
http://health.groups.yahoo.com/group/AutismBehaviorProblems
http://health.groups.yahoo.com/group/autismaba
http://health.groups.yahoo.com/group/EnzymesandAutism
http://health.groups.yahoo.com/group/chelatingkids2
http://health.groups.yahoo.com/group/Autism-Mercury
http://health.groups.yahoo.com/group/DTT-NET
http://health.groups.yahoo.com/group/abmd
http://health.groups.yahoo.com/group/NIDS
http://health.groups.yahoo.com/group/abaparents
http://health.groups.yahoo.com/group/communicating

http://health.groups.yahoo.com/group/VerbalBehavior

http://health.groups.yahoo.com/group/AutismNCD

http://health.groups.yahoo.com/group/ANDI-ADI

http://groups.yahoo.com/group/EOHarm

http://health.groups.yahoo.com/group/Floortime

http://health.groups.yahoo.com/group/pecanbread

http://health.groups.yahoo.com/group/GFCFrecipes

http://health.groups.yahoo.com/group/Latetalkers

http://health.groups.yahoo.com/group/AspergersSupport

http://health.groups.yahoo.com/group/autismnet

http://health.groups.yahoo.com/group/fam-girls-autism

http://health.groups.yahoo.com/group/autism_insurance_information

http://health.groups.yahoo.com/group/autismfamilycircle

http://health.groups.yahoo.com/group/autism_support_group

http://health.groups.yahoo.com/group/Autism-Lead

http://health.groups.yahoo.com/group/parenting_autism

http://groups.yahoo.com/group/FOODALLERGYKITCHEN

http://in.groups.yahoo.com/group/AutismIndia

http://listserv.icors.org/scripts/wa-icors.exe?A0=ASPERGER

http://listserv.icors.org/scripts/wa-icors.exe?A0=CEL-KIDS

http://listserv.icors.org/scripts/wa-icors.exe?A0=CELIAC

http://www.udel.edu/bkirby/asperger

http://forums.delphiforums.com/hfasd/start

http://forums.delphiforums.com/celiac

Information on Autism Spectrum Disorders, Celiac Disease, Diets, and Interventions

Autistic Spectrum Disorders

http://www.autismspeaks.org

http://www.maapservices.org
http://www.autism-society.org/site/PageServer
http://www.autismdigest.com
http://www.autismhelp.info/main.htm
http://www.asno.org/products.htm#3
http://childbrain.com
http://www.generationrescue.org
http://www.autismtreatmentcenter.org/archives/2003/topicf14d.html
http://www.templegrandin.com
http://www.breakingtheviciouscycle.info/news/autism_one_radio.htm
http://www.theautismperspective.org
http://www.enabling.org/ia/celiac/aut/vitam-b6.html
http://www.nationalautismassociation.org
http://www.isn.net/~jypsy
http://www.surfershealing.com
http://rdiconnect.com
http://www.sandbox-learning.com
http://www.ponderethereal.com/index.php/2005/03/2648
http://www.autismndi.com
http://www.normalfilms.com
http://www.rdos.net/eng/Aspie-quiz.php
http://www.autismtoday.com
http://www.wrightslaw.com/info/autism.index.htm
http://www.foodb.com
http://www.greenpeople.org/healthfood.htm
http://www.nationalautismassociation.org/helpinghand.php
http://www.jkp.com
http://www.cafepress.com/aspieland
http://www.tonyattwood.com.au
http://www.usautism.org/about_us.htm
http://www.talkaboutcuringautism.org

http://www.autism.com
http://www.autism.com/ari/atec/atec-online.htm
http://www.bbbautism.com/diagnostics_psychobabble.htm
http://www.canadianautism.com
http://www.autism-india.org
http://health.groups.yahoo.com/group/GFCFAustralia
http://health.groups.yahoo.com/group/GFCFkidsUK

Celiac Disease and Diet Information

http://www.gfcfdiet.com
http://www.kidswithfoodallergies.org
http://www.celiac.org
http://www.specialfoods.com
http://www.specialeats.com
http://capelife.org/DietaryIntervention.html
http://www.paleodiet.com/autism
http://www.autism-diet.com
http://www.gluten-free.org
http://www.glutenfree.com
http://www.gflinks.com
http://www.livingwithout.com
http://autismshare.com
http://www.glutenfreedrugs.com
http://www.csaceliacs.org
http://www.celiac.ca/EnglishCCA/ccaenglish.html
http://www.glutenfreeholidays.com
http://www.enabling.org/ia/celiac/groups/groupsin.html
http://www.bakeriesworld.com/glutenfree.html
http://bedrokcommunity.org/index.html
http://coeliac.org.uk/food_business/media_opportunities/145.asp
http://www.celiachealth.org/pdf/GlutenFreeDietGuideWeb.pdf

http://www.jackshouse.org/Resources.aspx

http://www.celiaccentral.org (Raising Our Celiac Kids)

http://www.celiac.com/articles/563/1/ROCK-Raising-Our-Celiac-
Kids---National-Celiac-Disease-Support-Group/Page1.html

http://www.celiac.com/categories/Celiac-Disease-%26amp%3B-Kids-
by-Danna-Korn

Interventions

http://www.danasview.net

Applied Behavior Analysis (ABA)

http://www.abainternational.org

http://www.behavior.org/autism

Discrete Trial Teaching (DTT)

http://www.ehow.com/how_2088308_use-dtt-treat-autism.html

Neurofeedback

http://www.eegspectrum.com

http://www.eeginfo.com/info_what.htm

http://www.aboutneurofeedback.com

http://www.isnr.org

Listening Therapy

http://www.tomatis-group.com

http://www.drguyberard.com

http://www.soundlistening.com

http://www.tuneyourears.com/html/Listening_Therapy/intro.php

http://www.toolsforwellness.com/ce301.html

Yeast
http://www.healing-arts.org/children/antifungal.htm
http://bedrokcommunity.org/index.html
http://danasview.net/yeast.htm
http://www.adhdrelief.com/CandidaTest.html
http://www.candidapage.com

Enzymes and Supplements
http://www.enzymestuff.com/conditionpdd.htm
http://www.autismcoach.com/enzyme_survey.htm
http://www.autismcoach.com/Supplements.htm
http://www.usprobiotics.org

B Vitamins
http://www.howstuffworks.com/vitamin-b.htm
http://www.holistichealthtopics.com/HMG/Bvitamin.html
http://www.doctoryourself.com/bvitamins.html
http://www.enabling.org/ia/celiac/aut/vitam-b6.html
http://www.autism.org/vitb6.html

Allergens
http://www.foodallergy.org
http://www.foodallergy.org/allergens/index.html
http://www.allergen.org/Allergen.aspx
http://allergyadvisor.com/hidden.htm

Chelation
http://www.healing-arts.org/children/holmes.htm
http://www.chelationwatch.org

Hyperbaric Oxygen Therapy (HBOT)

http://www.hbotreatment.com/Autism.htm

http://www.healing-arts.org/children/hyperbaric.htm

Helpful Information on Various Disabilities and Services

http://www.betterhealthusa.com/public/160.cfm

http://www.dsc.ucsf.edu/main.php

http://www.uniquelygifted.org

http://www.healthboards.com/boards/index.php

http://www.kidfoundation.org/what/index.html

http://www.magazines.com/ncom/mag?id=3186382520190&mid=0000006297

http://www.allkindsofminds.org

http://www.generationrescue.org/index2.html

http://www.ataccess.org/rresources/CARTbiblio.html

http://www.add.org

http://www.disabilities-r-us.com

http://www.disabilityresources.org

http://www.enablelink.org

http://www.eparent.com

http://www.medicinenet.com/script/main/hp.asp

http://www.healthyplace.com

http://www.familyvillage.wisc.edu/index.htmlx

http://www.kidneeds.com

http://kidshealth.org/parent

http://www3.niaid.nih.gov

http://www.curesearch.org

http://www.easterseals.com/site/PageServer

http://www.disabledstudent.net

http://www.our-kids.org
http://www.specialchild.com/index.html
http://parentpals.com/gossamer/pages
http://www.fcsn.org
http://nmha.org
http://www.ucp.org
http://national.unitedway.org
http://www.patientcenters.com
http://www.clanthompson.com/news_sample.php3
http://j.webring.com/hub?ring=celiac
http://www.dbsalliance.org
http://specialchild.com/index.html
http://ideallives.com
http://digestive.niddk.nih.gov/ddiseases/a-z.asp
http://www.specialneeds.com

These two websites are good places to start looking for help in locating services: the National Dissemination Center for Children with Disabilities (http://www.nichcy.org) and the Autism Research Institute (http://www.autism.com/treatable/index.htm).

For other countries check the United Nations website for assistance: (http://www.un.org/disabilities/countries.asp?navid=12&pid=166).

You might want to contact your state's, province's, or country's education department to have them point you in the right direction to obtain services to assist your child. For other countries, contact the agencies listed below for further laws, regulations, and services that can help support your child.

Locate your state's, province's, or country's name below and further investigate the services available to you and your family.

United States

Alabama: http://www.alsde.edu/html/sections/section_detail.asp?section
=65&footer=sections

Alaska: http://www.hss.state.ak.us/gcdse

Arizona: http://www.arizonaautism.org

Arkansas: http://arksped.k12.ar.us

California: http://www.cde.ca.gov/sp/se/sr

Colorado: http://www.cde.state.co.us/index_special.htm

Connecticut: http://www.state.ct.us/sde/deps/special

Delaware: http://www.doe.state.de.us/programs/specialed

Hawaii: http://doe.k12.hi.us/specialeducation/spedisitforyourchild.htm

Kansas: http://www.kansped.org/

Kentucky: http://www.education.ky.gov/KDE/Default.htm

Louisiana: http://www.doe.state.la.us/lde/specialp/home.html

Maryland: http://www.marylandpublicschools.org/MSDE/divisions/
earlyinterv

Mississippi: http://www.mde.k12.ms.us/special_education

Montana: http://www.opi.state.mt.us/SpecEd

Nebraska: http://www.nde.state.ne.us/SPED/iepproj/index.html

New Hampshire: http://www.ed.state.nh.us/education/doe/
organization/instruction/bose.htm

New Jersey: http://www.nj.gov/njded/specialed

New Mexico: http://www.ped.state.nm.us/seo

North Carolina: http://www.ncpublicschools.org/ec

North Dakota: http://www.dpi.state.nd.us/speced/index.shtm

Ohio: http://www.ode.state.oh.us/exceptional_children/children_with_
disabilities

Oklahoma: http://se.sde.state.ok.us/ses

Oregon: http://bluebook.state.or.us/education/specialed/specialed.htm

Pennsylvania: http://www.pde.state.pa.us/special_edu/site/default.asp

South Carolina: http://www.myscschools.com/offices/ec

South Dakota: http://doe.sd.gov/oess
Tennessee: http://www.state.tn.us/education/speced
Texas: http://www.tea.state.tx.us/special.ed
Utah: http://www.usoe.k12.ut.us/sars
Vermont: http://www.state.vt.us/educ/new/html/pgm_sped.html
Virginia: http://www.pen.k12.va.us/VDOE/sess
Washington: http://www.k12.wa.us/SpecialEd/publications.aspx
West Virginia: http://wvde.state.wv.us/ose
Wisconsin: http://www.dpi.state.wi.us/dpi/dlsea/een
Wyoming: http://www.k12.wy.us/ao/sp/programs/speced.asp

Canada

Check these sites and then search for your province, or check the
province-specific sites below: http://www.edu.gov.on.ca/eng/relsites/
oth_prov.html or http://www.greenwoodmfrc.ca/english/cis/educa-
tion/special_needs_e.htm

Alberta: http://education.alberta.ca/admin/special.aspx
British Columbia: http://www.gov.bc.ca/themes/education_literacy/
special_education.html
Manitoba: http://www.edu.gov.mb.ca/k12/specedu/index.html
New Brunswick: http://www.inclusiveeducation.ca/learn/publications.
asp
Northwest Territories: http://www.ece.gov.nt.ca
Nova Scotia: http://www.ednet.ns.ca/pdfdocs/studentsvcs/specialed/
speceng.pdf
Nunavut: http://www.gov.nu.ca/education
Ontario: http://www.edu.gov.on.ca/eng/general/elemsec/speced/
ontario.html
Prince Edward Island: http://www.gov.pe.ca/educ/index.
php3?number= 76715

Quebec: http://www.mels.gouv.qc.ca/gr-pub/menu-curricu-a.htm#table

Saskatchewan: http://www.sasked.gov.sk.ca/branches/curr/special_ed/seindex.shtml

Yukon: http://www.education.gov.yk.ca

Other Countries

Australia: http://www.answd.org

Austria: http://www.european-agency.org/site/national_pages/austria

Belgium/Flemish: http://www.european-agency.org/site/national_pages/belgium_flemish

Belgium/French: http://www.european-agency.org/site/national_pages/belgium_french

China: http://www.china.org.cn/english/features/38282.htm

Cyprus: http://www.european-agency.org/site/national_pages/cyprus/index.html

Czech Republic: http://www.european-agency.org/site/national_pages/czech_republic

Denmark: http://www.european-agency.org/site/national_pages/denmark

Estonia: http://www.european-agency.org/site/national_pages/estonia

Finland: http://www.european-agency.org/site/national_pages/finland

France: http://www.european-agency.org/site/national_pages/france

Germany: http://www.european-agency.org/site/national_pages/germany

Greece: http://www.european-agency.org/site/national_pages/greece

Hungary: http://www.european-agency.org/site/national_pages/hungary

Iceland: http://www.european-agency.org/site/national_pages/iceland

India: http://www.autismindia.com

Ireland: http://www.european-agency.org/site/national_pages/ireland

Italy: http://www.european-agency.org/site/national_pages/italy

Japan: http://www.education-in-japan.info/sub207.html

Latvia: http://www.european-agency.org/site/national_pages/latvia

Lithuania: http://www.european-agency.org/site/national_pages/lithuania

Luxembourg: http://www.european-agency.org/site/national_pages/
luxembourg

Malta: http://www.european-agency.org/site/national_pages/malta

Netherlands: http://www.european-agency.org/site/national_pages/
netherlands or http://www.landelijknetwerkautisme.nl

New Zealand: http://www.minedu.govt.nz

Norway: http://www.european-agency.org/site/national_pages/norway

Philippines: http://www.deped.gov.ph/quicklinks/quicklinks2.asp?id=34

Poland: http://www.european-agency.org/site/national_pages/poland

Portugal: http://www.european-agency.org/site/national_pages/portugal

South Africa: http://www.info.gov.za/whitepapers/2001/educ6.pdf

Spain: http://www.european-agency.org/site/national_pages/spain

Sweden: http://www.european-agency.org/site/national_pages/sweden/
index.html

Switzerland: http://www.european-agency.org/site/national_pages/
switzerland

UK/Scotland: http://www.european-agency.org/site/national_pages/
united_kingdom/index_scotland.html

UK/Wales: http://www.european-agency.org/site/national_pages/
united_kingdom/index_wales.html

❧ Index ❦

⁂ About the Author ⁂

Barrie Silberberg has a bachelor of arts degree in liberal studies (education) and a multiple subjects teaching credential from California State University, Northridge, with postgraduate work in regular and special education. Barrie's most important job is being a Stay-at-Home-Mom (SAHM) to her two children and spending a lot of her free time volunteering at her children's schools and for charities that are important to her. She works part-time freelance writing, teaching American Sign Language, speaking at GFCF seminars, and is also a job counselor with the State of California, assisting individuals who have disabilities. Her family is a foster family for abandoned kittens, and she also shares her home with a dog and three cats.

31901046127710